Camping and DASH Diet Cookbook 2 Books in 1

Quick & Easy Recipes for Campers and DASH Diet Followers

By

Alvin Ray

Table of Contents

Book 1: Camping Cookbook

Easy and Scrumptious Recipes to Cook in Campfire and Enjoy the Beauty of Nature

Introduction

When it comes to spending the night at the campfire, a feeling of nostalgia occurs to see who will cook the finest marshmallow. Unfortunately, by the second day in a row of hot, cold dogs and restful dinners, this warm, flannel-coated feeling appears to disappear. Over the years, outdoor explorers have derived many strategies to use a campfire to prepare meals. Others are more complex than most, of course. E.g., many hiking and camping trips would probably not need you to create a roasting spit (unless you feel a little overenthusiastic).

Using immediate straight heat is the simplest method for cooking over a campfire. There are two approaches to do this. The 1st, the hoax of old boy scouts, is to individually cover food products in foil made of aluminum and put them on burning/hot coals. It needs constant testing, but for meals that required high heat, it is very efficient. The second strategy is literally to put a grill over an outdoor fire and cook your food in the backyard as you would. The fire's fumes from this route are less immediate, so cooking would usually be a bit lengthier.

You'll need the pots and saucepans for soups, stews, and pasta. Just generate the fire to cook them, let it demise down to the burning coals, and position the saucepan or pot over them. The trick to this approach is to manage the amount and intensity of hot coal since heat may become volatile pretty easily. The good thing is that cooking at the campsite is just as simple as a kitchen range usage once you've got that down.

Camping is a bit more critical than home cooking, so you can't order pizza if something goes wrong. If you begin cooking at the campsite, a little effort in your meal planning will go a long way. Your recipes would not only come out better; they would be simpler to carry out. Organize each meal and snack ahead of the camping trip to ensure that you don't burn through your food or get stranded consuming breakfast chips on the first night. Based on how you're camping, how the plan would look will differ significantly.

Chapter 1: Essentials for Camp-site Cooking

Undoubtedly, consuming nutritious food outdoors is one of the greatest parts of camping. It isn't that complicated with a little planning, imagination and the necessary equipment to make gourmet meals when cooking in the open. Few people say that camping can be stressful and challenging and particularly strain the food situation. Typically, it's easier to cook food when you camp as conveniently as possible. To secure you and your friends, discourage the usage of perishable food items and always implement the requisite hygiene procedures.

1.1Kitchen Essentials Checklist at Camping

Producing gourmet meals while cooking in the outdoors just isn't that difficult with a little preparation, creativity, and the right equipment. Eating good food outside is one of the best aspects of camping. In a futuristic society, you'd reach your camping site with a schedule about what you're planning to eat while you're there, and just be ready to set fire to get it started. Afterward, you should only eat and relax.

1. Camping stove

A camping stove is an important piece of equipment if you are contemplating cooking on your next camping trip. A camping stove for certain cooking types will be required, whether it is a singular or dual burner, cantilevered or table-top.

Safety is still a concern while cooking, so it's important to take all the appropriate precautions. If you are camping in tents, caravan or motorhome, it's important not to cook in the unit because of the possible fire danger. Also, poor ventilation can contribute to a build-up of toxic carbon monoxide.

2. Cool-box

For keeping the food fresh, milk chilled, and beverages cooled, cool boxes are important. Present in a range of forms, sizes, shapes, and cool boxes are ideal for avoiding things from spoiling off. If space is a priority when packing, cool bags are a useful, space-saving alternative.

3. Camping stove gas

If you do not have any fuel to start it up, there is no point in keeping a camping stove. Different stoves need various fuel types, but it's safe and convenient to use butane (generally in a blue high-pressure cylinder) or propane (in a red cylinder).

As it is safe and quickly portable, gas is a great complement for cooking fuel. Have a glance at our guide to gas and liquid fuels before using camping petrol.

4. Dinnerware

It might sound like a given, but it's simple to overlook that you may need to eat and drink something. Since it is safer for the atmosphere than to use single-use paper plates and disposable cutlery, it is worth investing in any reusable dinnerware. Here is what you would need:

- Plates
- Bowls
- Cups
- Mugs
- Forks and knives
- Teaspoons and spoons
- Dishes for Serving

5. Pots and pans for camping

You will need certain utensils to cook your meals, whether it's unique camping kitchen appliances or home-made cookware. On the market, there is a broad range of pots and pans available. Custom camping cookware is generally lighter, more durable and easy to carry. If you plan to cook large quantities for many people, it is necessary to note to carry larger utensils.

6. Camping kettle

Packing a kettle can help you have a cup of tea or coffee or cook some pasta or rice. There are many camping kettles on the deal, such as aluminum and stainless steel, as well as rapidly-packable folding kettles. If you're new to camping and have decided to book onto a pitch with electricity, any kettle rated at about 2kw or less will do the job.

7. Cooking utensils

No matter which recipe you are trying, you will, at some stage, require knives for slicing, wooden spoons for mixing and spatulas for tossing. Here is a rundown of what you would need:

- Wooden spoon
- Large spoons

- Tongs
- Spatula
- Whisk
- Sharp knife
- Chopping board

8. Water container

It is a concern of comfort to have a complete bottle of water. To refill the container and then use the provision each time you need it, use a tap at your camping site. From most outdoor stores, you can purchase foldable water containers and those with taps, which are simple to pack, move and use.

9. First aid kit

Whenever it comes to camping, protection always comes first. A small first aid kit is important for every camping trip. When cooking food, burns and cuts are fairly normal, and plasters and bandages may be very helpful. Here's a list of what you need in the kit:

· A variety of plasters

- Disposable sterile gloves
- A variety of bandages
- Tweezers
- Scissors
- Wipes for cleaning
- Thermometer
- Sticky tape
- Antiseptic cream
- Pain relievers

10. Folding toaster for camping

Affordable, filling and convenient, toast is an excellent camping meal to eat. There's no reason to carry the toaster with you from home if you have a foldable camping toaster. It's easy, healthy and great to cook with a camping toaster toasting bread, breakfast sandwiches, and teacakes and melting the cheese in your toast.

11. Table camping

You bought all the ingredients, brought all the camping equipment for cooking with you, accompanied a recipe, served it on plates, but where are you planning to eat it? Gather your family or mates around the camping table and make mealtime a shared experience. Camping tables can adapt too; just use the table to arrange a board game or glean everybody round for a game of cards.

12. Bin bags

A clean camp is a pleasant camp. Put all the garbage in huge bags and leave your campsite's area clean and clear; this would decrease the likelihood of predators having an interest and improve the confidence of all in the camp. The camping code of "leave no trace" is crucial to keep in mind, so you can do your hardest to end up leaving your pitch in the same condition as you find it in.

13. Washing up equipment

A healthy routine to fall into is to keep the pitch tidy. Don't encourage washing up to sit around, use the abundant washing facilities and have a talk with your fellow campers whilst you're at it. It's also a perfect meeting spot. If you don't have the essentials for cleaning up the equipment, the cookware can get dirty. Here is what you would need:

- Washing up liquid
- Towels
- Scouring pad
- Sponge
- Dish-cloth

14. Butterfly Can opener

There are few things more tedious than getting a Can but no Can opener or a bottle with no bottle opener while camping in a secluded place. None of these problems would be a challenge if you remember to carry your butterfly can opener, and you're guaranteed to be a famous part of the camp.

15. Storage of food

You would maintain your food balanced and your atmosphere orderly by using a range of containers. By putting them chilled in Tupperware in your cool box, putting your surplus food in containers and reusing it the next day, keep your ingredients new. Sheets of beeswax will even help keep food fresh if you don't have any containers.

16. The chimney starter

This foldable compact chimney can make the coal burn in moments without the need for harmful burning lighter fluid, extremely great while using charcoals.

17. Portable grill

While most campsites have campfires with grates, their state may be less than enticing. It is possible to position this portable grill on top of the campground grill (with collapsing legs) or use it on its own (when free-standing). If free camping on public grounds, where there are no grill grates that cover fire pits, this may be especially helpful.

18. Thermometer with quick-Reading

Knowing the precise condition of a slice of meat or the Dutch oven's interior condition may be really useful when you're just starting to cook outside. It's easier to know unless you evolve the senses to go through intuition. A perfect method to take a guess as the steak is done cooking or not is this probe thermometer.

You can actually get away without one if you are new to camping, but it's certainly the key to make things very pleasant.

19. Cast Iron skillet with a lid

This is the camp kitchen MVP. On a camp burner, over a campfire, or snuggled in a bed of charcoal, cast iron may be used. It has a structure that is inherently non-stick, superior heat preservation and is essentially indestructible.

20. Non-Stick skillet

It is debatable whether or not this is a "necessary" component of camp cooking equipment. Without it, you should get by. But whether you prepare scrambled eggs, pancakes, tuna, or

something else that's sensitive, there's no substitution for a decent skillet that doesn't stick. This skillet would last for years if paired with a fitting silicone or wooden spatula.

21. Dutch oven

One of the most useful items of camp cookware that you will own is a Dutch oven. If you can picture it, you can actually make it in a Dutch oven. Sauté, steam, boil, roast, and bake. A flat rim lid helps you to mount charcoals on top, while underneath, you can nestle coals with support legs on the bottom.

22. Egg Holder

There are a lot of dubious, almost gimmicky camping products out there, but it's actually worth a plastic egg holder. Before we planned to have one of these, we missed a lot of good eggs.

23. Steramine

After cleaning your dishes, to disinfect against bacteria and viruses, add one of these tablets to your rinse bucket. It's more powerful than old-fashioned chlorine, and on the skin, it's much gentler.

1.2 Food Hacks for Camping

There is nothing like dreaming on a pleasant summer night underneath the stars next to a couple of your friends. Camping is a common year-round practice, but it acts as a very enjoyable getaway while the trails are open, the sun shines, the animals have been out, and the flowers are in bloom throughout the spring or summer. Few people claim that camping can be exhausting and difficult, and they stress about the situation of food most notably. No need to panic; if you're a camping beginner or a camping veteran, here are some simple and convenient outdoor food hacks to make you sound like a professional backcountry cook under no time.

Create pancakes or eggs using empty condiment bottles

Up cycle your used dressing bottles for sauces or salads and keep those for the upcoming camping trip. Load them with the batter of pancake (to conveniently squeeze on the campfire grill after washing them out, of course). Or, on the Track towards the campsite, prevent cracking your eggs by whipping a dozen together and storing them in ketchup bottles to produce scrambled eggs in the morning. You may even prepare scrambled eggs or tasty omelets in any bag to carry with you in advance. Utilize water bottles or Mason jars if you do not have any vacant condiment bottles.

Make meals a waft with the help of foil packs.

Conceivably the simplest dining mess-free camping hack is by making and preparing your meals in the foil. Cover the meat, vegetables and seasonings and put them on the hot coals or on a campfire grate until cooked completely. To try with your grilled meat, give a chance to a 'baked' potato. You could cover up your buttered bread and cheese and make a melted grilled cheese for a simpler meal which everyone will enjoy. This way, you can also make any sweet dishes. In order to avoid burning yourself when you remove them, make sure you have some extensive grilling tongs.

Use skewers apart from marshmallows.

Though s'mores are practically a necessity for every camping trip, roasting sticks can also be used to prepare other foods. Take refrigerated biscuits with you and cover them across the stick to cook over the fire. By trying to cover them with some crescent roll dough, alter your hotdog into flavorful pigs in a blanket. Or to get everything nice and gooey over the fire, for a sweet delicacy by busting a frozen cinnamon roll at the end. Using REI's trick to transform your recycled bottle of water into a lightweight rolling pin to cook some dough if you want to get extra fancy.

Muffins and much more in the peels of orange

For your daily dose of vitamin C, pack a bag of oranges. Cut the orange in half and use the dried peels to make muffins for a simple camping food hack once you're done eating (or drinking your fresh juice). You can blend your own batter of orange peels in a jar and keep it cold. Wrap your loaded oranges in the foil and put them in the burning coals for approximately 10 to 15 minutes.

Plan for some nutritious treats to remain full during meals once you've geared up the food hacks for camping or hiking. Make some no-bake hash of peanut butter snack bites (no refrigeration required) snacks or paleo cooked nuts to wrap along with the hikes.

Tic Tac box for spices

Food for camping does not have to be boring! To bring more flavor to your meals, take along any of your favorite spices. With the herbs and seasoning, simple ole camping food recipes can be changed. A bit of fried chicken or a bit of chickpea is all right. In the mix, add some curry powder, and camping food just got a lot more enticing. Well, there are fantastic herbs and spices, but they're not always effective. And that's where empty packets/boxes of Tic Tac certainly be useful. With the built-in sprinkling feature to boot, they are lightweight and secure. It was as if they had been made for traveling. By covering all ends with a lighter, you may use a straw as well. Chop off one of the edges of the straw with scissors or a knife until you are about to use the spice, or just spill out the seasoning from the Tic Tac box.

Drop the pasta at home

Pasta is an outdoor adventurer's mate. It's an easy option to get on the hiking trail with carbs that are much needed. Pasta preparation, though may not be the most efficient. Your setup is minimal while you're camping, and you don't have the option of waiting 20-30 minutes for the pasta to prepare on a one-speed burner. That is where it comes out useful for quinoa. It's much healthier, ready in minutes, and needs even less water. Quinoa, a carbohydrate targeted by a camper.

On the go, Eggs

Eggs are an important meal for a lot of people. A big box of eggs will take up the bulk of the room. Contrary, eggs last for a long period of time. So, crack up a dozen eggs while you leave home and transfer them to a big plastic bottle. When it's preparation time, you should then spill them out. When you pour the eggs into the bottle, draw a line on the bottle after every egg you add, another handy technique. Now, you know just how many eggs you are dealing with while you are preparing. If you're at a big breakfast party, you don't want to waste the day cooking. Only carry a muffin tray with you and smash the eggs into the cubes. You will prepare 12 eggs all together on a grill or on a campfire. Maybe you've ended up saving half a day of work.

Not only for beer

On the camping holiday, most people would carry a small cardboard six-pack tray for them. But beer isn't really that is good for that portion tray. They're perfect for carrying your important kitchen items as well. Six ideal little holders for napkins, plastic utensils and condiments and you just thought that it was compostable junk.

Tinfoil is your partner.

Cooking a camping food needs a decent stove for camping. Right? Wrong. Having a little fire, covering the food in tin foil and softly throwing it in the fire to heat it up is a simple way to cook food. Now that is actually cooking for survival.

Fat is your partner too.

It may be daunting to know what food resources to carry while you are departing your base for a hard day of workout. Just note, fat is a friend of yours. The absorption of fats is half as sluggish as carbohydrates. For longer, this would make you fuller. So, bring those nuts, peanuts, cashews, avocados, and dark chocolate for you. Healthy fats for longer use means more energy.

Iced water, a box of cold cooler

It's always great to have a couple of extra bottles of water for the trip. You may find them interesting in more respects than one, though. Overnight, ice a few bottles and install them as temporary cooler bags to the cooler box. You not only have freezing cold water but maybe a couple of cold drinks as well.

Toasted marshmallows for adults

Marshmallows that are toasted are delightful. For all camping trip experiences, they are a must-have. Nevertheless, this adult camping meal hack adds a different level to s'mores. Dip your marshmallow into a cup of Bailey's after you toast it. Don't put it into consideration; just do it. It's yummy.

On the go, pancakes

Instant oatmeal is fine, but a much more spectacular dish to serve is campfire pancakes. Make your pancake batter, spill it into a Ziploc bag, and seal it (it can be as plain or fancy as you wish). Place it in a refrigerator (or put a lunchbox with an ice pack in it) if you're willing to. Cut off the bottom corners of the bag when its pancake time and squeeze out the batter for each pancake into the heated pan. Bonus points if you can turn the pancake without getting confused.

Bags for Coffee

This hack is for you if you'd like a cup of morning joe to have your gears going. This is essentially a combination of DIY coffee and tea. Place one serving of ground coffee into a coffee grinder before leaving home (or camp) and seal it with a string to make a tiny coffee pouch. Pop this bag into a mug much as you would for tea. Pour hot water into the mug after boiling water over a fire, and you're arranged with coffee.

One-pot breakfast

Toss in the vegetables of your preference and some sausage over a grill. Sauté them until completely cooked for a couple of minutes, and then pour in the eggs (from the bottle hack). The eggs can be scrambled or omelet type, cooked.

Cook with couscous

Productivity is the game's name for most campers living in the outdoors, and as far as food bases go, there will be few as effective as couscous. Couscous has a range of benefits over pasta and rice as an ingredient: it cooks quicker, needs no continuing attention or cooking nous to cook properly, and does not take as much water to prepare, which is a blessing in remote regions. Couscous is just as robust as its more ardent variants, which renders it easier to cut down on the time and energy you need for your next camping trip while preparing.

Pack up the use of bread

In certain homes, bread is the main food, but it does not always imply it resides in the camp kitchen. Compared to certain foods, bread loaves have a short lifetime, and in a truck filled to the hilt of freight bouncing along unsealed highways, if you are not vigilant, it will easily become an exotic species (or at least a somewhat misshapen one). Its ciabatta cousin is an unusual addition to a loaf of bread: wraps. Wrap bread remains fresh for way too long, is also more lightweight and robust than traditional bread, and is often easier to portion; for washing-averse campers, the concept of enclosing a portion of food in an edible package is often an appealing one. Wrap bread is the present that tends to offer as you camp or fly, whether it's an egg and ham burrito in the morning, a bacon and lettuce wrap for lunch or a chicken quesadilla for dinner.

Begin the day with oats from overnight

Overnight oats are simple both to prepare and consume, made popular by a generational fascination with mason jars. The idea of overnight oats is that sometimes in conjunction with plain yogurt, fruit and other more fanciful stuff, you layer dried oats and a splash of milk in a bowl and keep them overnight in the fridge to soak up the milk as well as other ingredients. Then, you get a well-rounded and full breakfast in the morning to start the day without additional cooking and cleaning.

Freeze foods to bring along with you

Cooking before you go requires both foresight and a lot of preparation, but the advantages are clear for those who get to camp late or who just can't be bothered to cook up a camp storm. You reduce the need for fresh ingredients that have to be stored or taking up tons of room in your fridge or cooler by making and storing meals before you go, although these meals will even help to maintain other items cold while frozen in containers. You can switch between freshly cooked and frozen meals if you travel from camp to camp on a regular or every-other-day basis (or actually camp for a prolonged period), or also hold the frozen meals as protection in case you are out of fresh food at an unexpected time.

1.3 Food Safety and Camping

There is no better way than picking up a few things and going out to your ideal camping place to explore the outdoors with family and friends or even alone. It is necessary, though, to ensure that the food and water you intend to use is healthy, whether taken from home or scavenged in the wilderness. The easiest way of making a camping trip goes wrong is to ignore food hygiene. Any vacation can be spoiled by food or water poisoning, which can also contribute to harmful and long-lasting medical problems that you can almost definitely regret.

It's generally better to make some food preparation you'll be doing as safe as possible while camping. In order to ensure the protection of yourself and the people involved in your party, stop utilizing perishable food products and always use the necessary hygiene procedures. However, the barbecue and cookouts are a favorite of the camping culture. For this purpose, while cooking in the natural surroundings, it is necessary to watch all the appropriate safety precautions for preparing food.

The need to practice proper food safety

If adequate safety measures are not taken, there are many harmful and disease-causing organisms that can and may contaminate the food and drink. More than 200 foodborne illnesses have been reported by microbiologists. Many of these infections are contagious and are caused by a combination of viruses, parasites, and bacteria. Hazardous substances and contaminants are also a big source of anxiety and may cause intense disease. The biggest threat for someone who braves the woods is the foodborne disease. For that purpose, the number one safety concern should be food hygiene and food safety.

More caution might be needed, depending on the place, time of year, and other variables. Also, contact municipal officials for any hazards of contamination that might be found in local water sources, as well as for any viruses that are likely to be borne by local wildlife. While enjoying wild game not cooked by a specialist, special caution should be taken. Until prior inspection by a certified food service official, hunters and others in a hunter's group are warned not to consume the wild game.

Keep cold food cold and hot food hot.

It is not necessary to overestimate the value of refrigeration. Over the decades, refrigeration has saved countless lives and is your first protection against food spoiling and inducing disease from microbes, insects, and other creatures. In the first lines of protection against foodborne disease is the propensity to chilled meats and other ingredients. Cold foods often need extra care and must at all times be held at or below 41 degrees Fahrenheit. Food can never be left out for longer than 2 hours, less than an hour if the weather is over 90 degrees F, at room / outdoor temperatures.

It is not very popular to take hot food camping because most hot food consumed outdoors is prepared on a camp stove or open fire, but it does not imply that you are not at risk. In the two-hour cycle following cooking, food cooked in the camp must be eaten or stored in a colder location.

Choose foods with little to no planning required.

It sounds gourmet to have a steak or stuffed chicken breast but may create more issues than its value. Canned or pre-packaged foods can make life around the camp simpler and safer. Try canned chicken instead of taking in fresh chicken. For dried noodles and dehydrated vegetables that need just hot water, bring the favorite soup mixes. There are several raw food alternatives that require immediate planning, and that will decrease the risks of unsafe handling.

The best means to be assured

The perfect way to guarantee that your food stays nutritious is to keep it cool. You have a number of choices when it comes to freezing food for camping. Certain choices are safer than others, but while camping, to conserve your food, there are a few simple-to-apply low temperatures.

Using a cooler for camping

Your first line of protection against foodborne diseases is a good quality, sealed camping cooler or traveling refrigerator. A cooler preserves cold air, which keeps the product from having contaminants, germs and other kinds of pollution.

As Ice Packs, use chilled water bottles

The use of ice packs or random ice cubes to freeze your camping cooler may be enticing. However, there is an option that is easier and more helpful: frozen bottles of water. You can preserve your food and beverages by using chilled water bottles without trying to create extra room for ice. Best of all, you may easily consume the water in the bottles while your food intake decreases and the storage requirements diminish. It's a smart way of maximizing the space of your bag, keep the strain off your trash-pack at a minimum, and decrease the overall number of variables that contribute to food contamination.

Eat meat below 40 ° F

When meat and other related items are frozen, they could be infected, and it is not advised to refreeze them. Foods not processed at 40 ° F or below may often not be cooked reliably sufficiently to be made healthy. And if you're sure you can sterilize infected food at home quickly, it's almost difficult to be sure it's healthy while cooking from a campfire or trying to set up your camping kitchen. Lunch meats are supposed to be consumed cold, and if you are a novice at cooking outside, it might be your best choice.

Cook meats appropriately

How to correctly cook meat when camping cooked meat must always be prepared with extra care while camping. It may be extremely risky to catch a foodborne disease when camping, as emergency treatment would always be harder to find than it will be at home. At 160 ° F, cook ground beef, lamb, pork, veal and related meats. It must be cooked to 165 ° F for hot dogs. Cook poultry to 165 degrees F. It must be cooked to 145 ° F for unground beef, pork, lamb and veal. Before carving or eating these meats, let them rest for 3 minutes. The menu can even contain the internal temperature at which the meat should be, whether you are using a recipe from a camping cookbook.

Much like the one you use at home, you ought to have a meat thermometer to measure the temperature of every meat listed in this section. In the center of the meat, place the thermometer and give it time to show a suitable temperature. Until and unless it is sterilized, do not extract the thermometer and use it. It may be a smart practice to get more than one meat thermometer.

Cross-contamination prevention while cooking

Even if you think all the required measures are followed, it only takes one error to transfer a hazardous pathogen or parasite from every surface to your food. Before going on to another task, please be mindful of the last thing you have handled or the last thing the object in your hand touched. Here are a few tips to better guarantee the avoidance of cross-contamination.

Get the hands washed.

Before and after touching meat, utensils, dishware or anything that touches food, use eco-friendly cleaner and wash your hands. Clean your hands before preparing and serving meals, and after consuming and cleaning up and between each food-handling activity.

Clean up the containers and utensils

It can be easy to overlook the cross-contamination dangers of careless utensil use, much like the meat thermometer we described above. Try to restrict a specific jar and/or food product to each utensil. Clean utensils that pass from one table to another, one food product to another, and so forth, just like you wash your hands at any juncture.

Have various utensils and containers for various foods

It is a smart practice while cooking to restrict each utensil to a particular type of food. You will not use the exact tool to turn the meat that you are using to mix a soup or stew, for instance. Similarly, do not put food on a tray or jar that has been in an earlier step of preparation that has seen a particular form of food or a food component. Try to keep the camping kitchen organizers in your compact camping kitchen with various cutting boards and utensils. Whenever an uncooked food product from a refrigerator has been pulled, no food can go back into the container.

Refrain from getting leftovers

What to do when camping with Leftover Food? Leftovers from every camping trip can always be prevented. And if you take all the right steps before you manage to get back home, there is still a chance of food going awry. Prospects are that the ice would be used up or melted by the end of your trip, and any bugs, insects, or parasites will have the full chance to reproduce, grow, and do all the nasty stuff they do. Your safest solution is to leave leftovers and to remove those you might have responsibly. Food processed at temperatures between 40 ° F and 140 ° F is at the greatest risk of bacterial growth. Wasting food, of course, is not ideal. Make sure to heat them properly to combat any bacteria or undesirable disease-causing bacteria if you have any leftovers that you don't want to throw out. At the camping site, do not toss away wasted food. This can draw harmful wildlife to other campers and pose a threat.

Safe water for consumption

For people outdoors, the opportunity to access clean water for drinking has long been an obstacle. Locations where polluted water occurs, have been assigned terrifying names by Native Americans. We have more solutions for washing and preserving water open to us today. Nevertheless, preventing water-borne illnesses and acquiring clean water is not something that can be approached easily.

Don't drink water from a natural source directly.

There is no need to drink straight from some river, stream, lake, or pond unless you are in a dire survival condition. There are purifiers for camping water, which may be helpful in an emergency scenario. It is still safer to carry the water you consume, though. If necessary, keep water purifiers for extreme emergencies.

Bring to drink your own Filtered Water.

The only way to be absolutely confident that the drinking water is pure and healthy is to bring clean water with you. Toxic contaminants, and the most insidious hazardous chemicals, will defeat even high-quality compact water purifiers. Any fair guarantee of protection and purity comes only with bottled water taken from the home.

Using water filtering and facilities for purification

The water purifying apparatus is a reasonable choice, as stated. The industry has a range of camping filtration systems and purifiers. If you choose to use one of these substitutes, make sure that it is of a good standard. The ideal, as mentioned, is to use filtered water from home. Filters and purifiers are, though, good choices in an emergency scenario. Our suggestion is to use them only as a supplement to your bottled water source.

Chapter 2: Cooking Over Campfire

Collating around a fireplace with family and friends to share a campfire-cooked meal is one of the best aspects of a camping trip. What might have been better than the sound of creaking wood and the scent of woodland dinner?

For more than a million years, humans have been cooking in the woods. Cooking and eating around the fire sounds normal and can be performed by everyone. After a day of exploring, several people have great memories of mushy toasted marshmallows melting in the mouths or their mom and dad serving up dripping healthy fish that they captured earlier that day. Cooking at a campfire makes it unique for a camping trip. Advanced camp stoves and customized cookware make the cooking job much easier.

2.1 Safe Cooking Tips at Campsite

The existence of open fires or stoves is one of the main causes of danger during camp cooking. Of course, where you are camping, you should always obey the guidelines and restrictions in place, particularly those that have to do with fire protection. Most campsites have fireplaces. Before cooking, please check that you recognize your campground fire rules.

Whether there is no fireplace and no stoves, make sure the fire is at least 15 feet off any tents, vegetation, cars, flammable items or branches overhanging. Create a rock surface fire as much as possible. Check for bare mineral soil if no rock is accessible.

Further are fire prevention tips for cooking at the campsite:

- Never let kids close to a stove or fire.
- Ensure everyone understands the universal fire protection protocol, like how to "stop, drop, and roll." flames, tents, cars and heat.
- If a compressed gas cylinder needs to be filled or a liquid bottle is replenished, cool the stove completely before deciding to do so.
- Clean all spills up instantly to reduce the chance of the fire spreading unintentionally by using flammable liquids such as starter fluid.
- Make sure that the tent is on a flat surface with a camp stove.
- Make sure that both tanks and hoses are not affected by using a stove. And tiny leaks can be

very harmful. To inspect all ties for leakage, use water and liquid soap.

- Do not leave a fire or unattended stove burning.
- To mitigate the chance of unintended ingestion, mark all flammable liquids.
- You always have at least one convenient oven mitt to treat hot things.
- Do have a water pail ready if the fire gets out of control.

Have the following in mind when it is time to put out the fire:

- If required, it's always thinkable to help the wood to burn completely into ash.
- Continue to throw water on the flames until it has drowned all the embers and ceases hissing.
- Stir with a shovel or a long branch to guarantee that anything previously on fire is moist and cool to the touch.
- Mix sand or dirt with the embers if you do not have enough water to drown the flames until all the stuff is cold for the touch.
- Stir continuously. When a fire is merely buried, it can always leave it smoldering underground, only to rise to the surface later and trigger a forest fire.
- Good thumb rule: if it's too hot to handle, it's too hot to be left unattended.

2.2 Techniques for Campfire Cooking

Advanced camp stoves and customized cookware make the cooking job much easier; however, nothing beats a meal prepared over the campfire's taste and appeal. Success in campfire cooking will inspire you more often to go camping.

Respect and warnings

Cooking over a campfire might be overlooked in days gone by. Today, with considerations about air quality, limited camping areas, and decreasing stocks of firewood in many camping sites, the liberty to cook over a campfire is a pleasure that requires the greatest caution and respect. Here are some significant factors:

Wood

Campfire cooking needs a clean-burning fire. Only dry, seasoned wood achieves this. It is pointless to strip green wood trees-your fire would be pungent, burn badly, and generate excessive pollution. It will need to be stocked in if dry wood is not obtainable. Firewood is supplied by many community campgrounds-calls ahead to see what is available.

Location of Fire

Before preparing a certain fire, pay heed to the ground. In situations where it is not possible to build your fire on a stone, one should make sure that the foundation of the fire is on dry mineral soil. There is a lot of time for a fire that burns all evening to burn through the soil's organic layer and will not be put out with a plain bucket of water. To avoid bruising the area with more fireplaces, use pre-existing fire pits if available.

The Wind

Any wind from medium to strong is dangerous. A forest fire can be ignited by the risk of flames getting away. The coals will also lessen more rapidly and offer far less cooking time. Any exterior fire will be out of the question if a significant wind shelter is inaccessible.

How to construct a cooking campfire?

The goal is to turn all the wood into coal at the same time. This provides a fire even without flames flying up to burn the food or darken the cookware. It also gives the coals the lengthiest cooking time.

Site preparation

- Choose at least 8' from bushes or any flammable fire site. Be sure the site doesn't overhang any tree branches.
- Using big rocks or green logs, end up making a U-shaped boundary. If logs are used, they will need to be wet periodically. If it's breezy, experience the wind from the back of the fire pit.
- Place a massive flat rock at the backside of the fire pit to make it act as a chimney. The 'rock of the chimney' will help direct the fumes up and away.

Build the Kindling

- With folded paper or tinder, fill the fire area.
- Lay kindling in layers over the paper, the alternating route with each layer. Use thin timber splits or a couple of dead branches. Do not place "teepee style" kindling down. With the kindling pile, the entire fire area should be filled.

- Set a water bucket near the area of the fire. To start your fire, beam the paper.

Generate the fire, level the coals.

- Add firewood when the kindling is incinerated. The timber should be as large as possible, all of same size. Use branches of hardwood if available. Divide wood equally over the bed of the fire.
- Use a stick to steer the coals to a greater level at the rear end and low degree at the front as quickly as the last flames die down, leaving mostly white coals. This gives you the equivalent of cooking settings for 'Hi',' Med' and 'Low'. Or, level the coals to your liking.
- Fixed the grill on stones or wet green logs to cook. Put food on the grill or in the cookware directly and start preparing your meal. A tiny spray bottle or sprinkle gun helps take down any malicious flames when cooking explicitly on the grill, caused mainly by food drippings.
- When the fire decreases, the coals are banked to get as much heat from them.
- Then add wood for the evening campfire after cooking. Dispel thoroughly and drench with water prior to removal. Turn the rocks into a bed of fire. If required the next day, it will be easy to reconstitute.

Fire-safe ovens and high-efficiency stoves for outdoor cooking

A solar oven is a great alternative if you can't have a campfire because of fire restrictions. All you need is sunlight, and without a flame, you can bake, boil, or steam. A camp stove with an insulated firebox is another option, such as the Firebox Nano, that provides low-emission, high-efficiency contained outdoor cooking fires.

Sun Oven: For camp cooking: In areas where fires are limited

- The power of the sun bakes, boils, or steams any kind of food.
- No fire is required! No fuel is required!
- Ideal for daily use in the backyard, for picnics, camping, or in the event of a power failure

Firebox stoves: For safe, enclosed, effective cooking fires

- Burns wood with a system of cross-feeding
- Super-efficient fuel utilization with very low emissions
- Suitable for outdoor camping, picnics and preparedness for emergencies

Clean Cooking Water for Campfire

You have several choices while preparing meals outdoors to ensure that your water is safe for cooking and drinking:

Use water, such as the drainpipe in a campground from a credible source of drinking water. These will be identified as potable sources of water by parks as well as other authorities.

Using water slabs or other food-grade containers, bring water into your campsite. At least one minute before actually using it for cooking, boil the water that is collected from every wilderness source. Boil water for at least three minutes if you're at elevations higher than 2,000 meters (6,562 feet).

Some useful tips for cooking food over a campfire

Prior to adding it to the pot, purify the cooking water with a credible backcountry filtration system.

Using the proper gear

When it refers to campfire meals, the options are infinite, but you must have the right instruments for the task to make tasty foods. For a cooking area, a grill grate is an ideal option. For boiling water, baking, or slow cooking, you may cook meat and vegetables straight on the grill or use it as a rack to carry pots and pans.

For campfire cooking, cast iron cookware is preferred since the dense metal absorbs heat easier and disburses it more equally. A cast-iron pot, pan, and a Dutch oven provide certain cast iron necessities. Do not forget utensils for stirring and serving, such as stainless-steel tongs and a long-handled spatula. Safety and cleaning equipment like grill gloves, a wire grill cleaner, and a digital meat thermometer may also be required.

Don't miss the foil of aluminum.

This multipurpose product can be used to cover cookware, cover fruits and vegetables directly in the coals for frying and create protein packages for gently cooking. You may also mold it in a pinch to form a simple pot or serving dish.

Do the meal preparation at home.

Do as much of the meal prep job as possible at home for fast cooking. When all your utensils are within easy reach, slicing and dicing meat and vegetables are easier at home. Place your ingredients in baskets for storage and bring them with you. To preserve freshness, place cold products such as meat and milk in a cooler filled with ice bricks. Alternatively, to hold it fresher for longer, vacuum seal the product at home.

Do not cook explicitly over the bare fire.

Burnt food is the one thing that cooking explicitly over the fire will do. The excessive heat characterizes your meat's exterior or cooks' dishes unequally, which is not just uncomfortable but also unsafe. In order to hold your cookware above the most extreme fire, wait until the coals are white-hot and use a cooking surface or stand.

Choose the right cooking technique.

There are several options to cook around a campfire, so depending on the dish you intend to produce, the cooking procedure and the cookware you need to carry with you. If you are hunting and planning to cook wild game, for low, slow cooking like braises or stews, carry along with your cast iron cookware. If you just want to grill some hot dogs or make s' mores, however, then a heavy cast-iron skillet doesn't need to be carried; a few long skewers or a grill are enough. Some campfire dishes, such as campfire baked potatoes or filled roasted apples, focus on directly dipping ingredients in the coals.

To dampen Flare-ups, use a spray bottle.

Sparks that may contribute to flare-ups can be quickly sparked by oil and grease splashes from cooking. The heat circulation in your cookfire may also be modified by flare-ups, allowing the food to cook unequally. Spray it with a few blasts of water from a spray bottle as soon as you see a wayward flame or ember to hold your campfire contained. In certain situations, eliminating frying items that are clumpy or prone to spill fat may be a safer option. If you have to fry the food, use a low-oil Dutch oven to avoid splatters from rising.

Have water and sand ready

If the wind kicks up or they're left exposed, campfires may easily get out of hand. Have a bucket of water and sand for each to drench and lessen the fires easily if they seem like they are growing.

Even to extinguish the fire when you are done, keep water and sand ready. Add water or sand to set the campfire out correctly before leaving, then use a long metal whisk to stir the flames. When the fire and coals are smothered and cold, begin this process.

Final thoughts

A perfect way to explore nature and to spend quality time with friends and family is to cook over a campfire. You should always search for more hints, techniques, and tasty wild game recipes if you usually spend time in the great outdoors and have a love of cooking.

Chapter 3: Delicious Recipes for Camping

There just isn't anything like dreaming below the stars and staying away from city life's daily grind. They don't label it "roughing it" for nothing, of course. Some aspects of the camping experience are less than enticing, and one of them could be the food. When you end up leaving your cook-top and oven back in the house, there's no denying that cooking gets quite a bit harder. Yet, there are several choices for making your trip even smoother these days because technology is on your side. You might notice that cooking over a fire is not as difficult as you thought, as long as you do some preparation and plan ahead. There's no need to make camping food confusing or dull! These delicious food ideas for camping can make trip planning simple and keep you looking forward to every meal.

3.1 Breakfast Recipes

1. Cast Iron Frittata

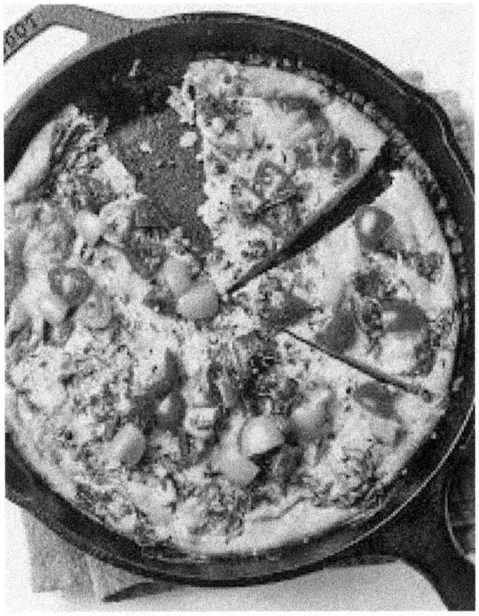

Serving: 4

Preparation time: 30 minutes

Nutritional values: 304kcal calories|6g carbohydrates|6g proteins|22g fat

Ingredients

- 8 eggs
- 1⁄2 cup of milk

- 1⁄2 teaspoon of sea salt
- 1⁄4 teaspoon of freshly ground pepper
- teaspoons of olive oil, cut,
- 1 shallot, thinly sliced
- 1 pint of cherry tomatoes, sliced in half
- 1⁄4 cup of basil, chopped
- 1⁄2 cup gruyere cheese shredded

Directions

1. For cooking, build a campfire or charcoal.
2. Beat the eggs, milk, salt and pepper together in a medium bowl until completely mixed. Set aside.
3. Heat 1 tablespoon of oil over medium heat in a 10 "skillet. Attach the shallot and sauté for 7-10 minutes, unless soft and browning start.
4. By lifting the campfire grater or shifting the skillet to the cold side of the grill, minimize the heat to medium-low. To the skillet, add the tomatoes, accompanied by the egg mix, basil, and cheese. Cover it with a lid cover. Scatter around the lid a few embers.
5. Cook for about 15 minutes until the frittata has ruffled and the eggs are set (check every 10 minutes to calculate change, use heatproof gloves or a cover lifter to remove the lid).
6. Serve and eat it with extra cheese and basil if needed.

2. Banana Bread Pancakes

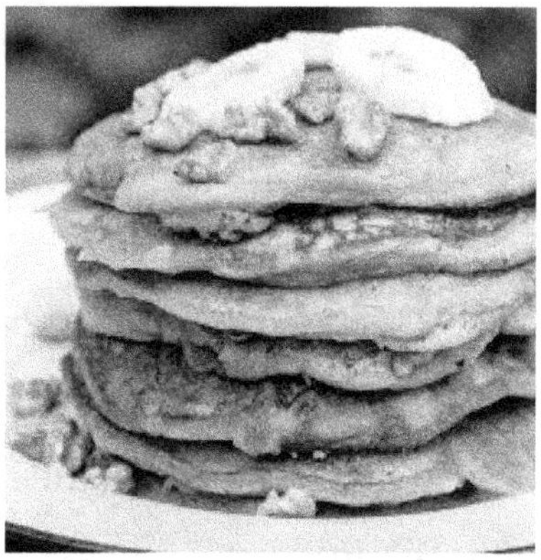

Serving: 16

Preparation time: 30 minutes

Nutritional values: 152kcal calories|9 g carbohydrates| 8g proteins|12g fat

Ingredients

- 3 bananas (the richer, the riper)
- 2 eggs
- 1 & 1⁄2 cup of whole milk
- 2 cups flour
- 1⁄4 cup of brown sugar
- 2 tsp of cinnamon
- 2 teaspoons of baking powder
- 1 teaspoon of salt
- 1 cup sliced walnuts (toasted if needed in a dry skillet)
- A pan for ghee, butter, or coconut oil

Directions

For Home

1. In a sealable bag or jar, add the flour, brown sugar, cinnamon, baking powder, and salt, and pack with the remaining ingredients.

At a Camp

1. In a medium bowl, put two bananas and mash thoroughly until moderately smooth with the back of a fork. Cram the egg in a mixture and add this to the milk. Beat together the banana, the egg and the milk until creamy.
2. Add the dry ingredients to the bowl and blend together with the wet ingredients until well mixed. Do not over-mix. Few little lumps are completely alright. You should add an optional 1/4 cup of milk if the batter is too thick.
3. Over medium-low to medium heat, place a nonstick pan or well-seasoned stainless-steel skillet on your burner. To coat the plate, add a gentle dab of ghee, butter, or coconut oil (particularly if cast iron is used!) and swirl. Onto the middle of the skillet, add 1⁄3 cup of the pancake batter and disperse some of the sliced walnuts on top. Cook before the top starts to bubble for a few

minutes, and the sides are set (2-3 minutes). Flip the pancake using a spatula and cook the other side until crispy.

4. For each pancake, repeat for the rest of the batter, adding more ghee or oil as required to the plate.
5. Stack the pancakes and line them with maple syrup or butter, sliced banana, and extra toasted walnuts for serving. Enjoy.

3. Perfect French Toast

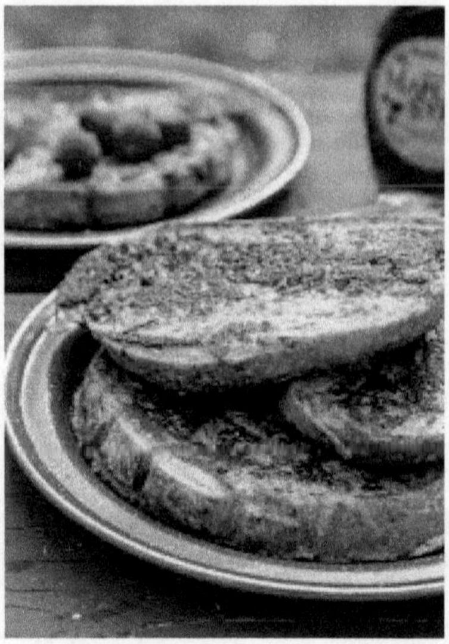

Serving: 8

Preparation: 30 minutes

Nutritional values: 275kcal calories| 125g carbohydrates|75g proteins| 89g fat

Ingredients

- 1/2 lb. loaf of bread
- Eggs
- 1 cup of milk
- tsp of butter, and plenty to scatter
- 1 teaspoon of cinnamon
- 1 teaspoon extract of vanilla, optional
- 1/4 teaspoon of nutmeg, optional

- tablespoons of butter for pan
- Top Maple Syrup & Berries

Directions

1. Cut the bread into slices 3/4-1" "thick.
2. First, beat the eggs in a big enough bowl to fit a slice of the bread. Then mix together milk, cinnamon, nutmeg, vanilla, and sugar, until fully blended.
3. Heat 4 teaspoons of butter over medium heat in a pan.
4. In the egg and milk mixture, dip a slice of bread and let it soak on each side for around 10 seconds. Let the excess trickle off, sprinkle additional sugar on each side, and then fry it on each side, approximately 3 minutes per side, in the skillet once get golden and crispy.
5. Repeat with the remainder loaf, adding more butter if required to the skillet.
6. Serve with maple syrup, fruit, and a hot coffee cup. Enjoy.

4. Avocado Toast Breakfast Sandwich

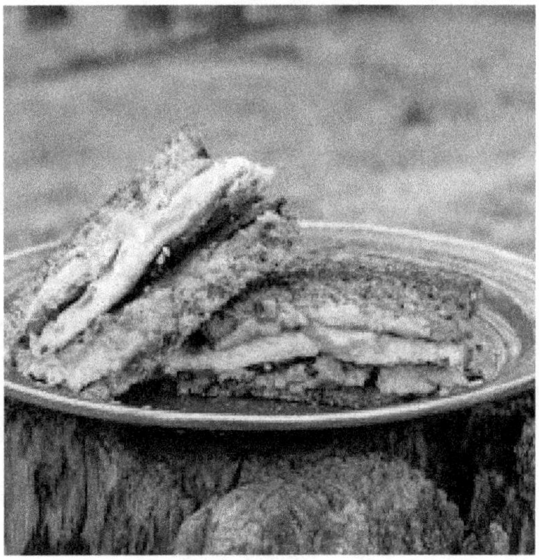

Serving: 1

Preparation time: 15 minutes

Nutritional values: 103kcal calories|8g carbohydrates|7g protiens|5g fat

Ingredients

- Bacon slices, sliced in half

- Bread slices
- 1 egg
- 1 avocado
- Salt + pepper
- Optional: a pinch of everything but the seasoning of the bagel

Directions

1. Set your campfire or camp stove with a cast-iron skillet over it. Put the bacon in the skillet and cook until crispy over medium-low heat, flipping periodically. Remove and place on a plate lined with a paper towel.
2. Toast/fry the bread in the pan, rotating so that all sides are browned after about a minute. Simply remove and set aside.
3. Add a bit more fat to the skillet if required. Crack the pan with an egg and prepare it to your taste.
4. Slice the avocado in half to assemble the sandwich, squirt out the center, and apply it on both slices of bread. Layer on one side the bacon, on the other side the egg, and season with salt & pepper.

5. Bacon, Egg and Avocado Sandwich

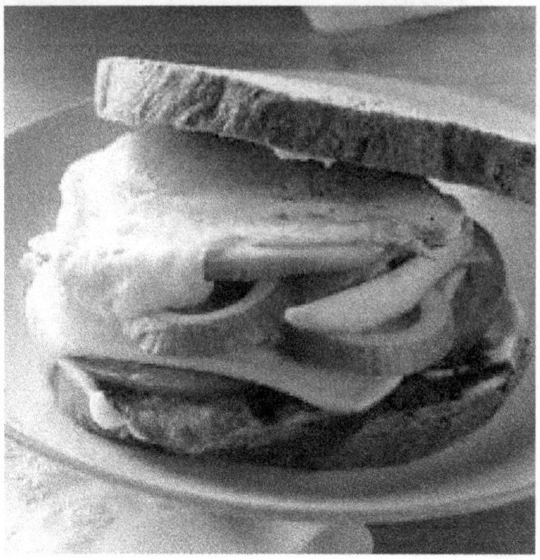

Serving: 2

Preparation time: 25 minutes

Nutritional values: 550 kcal calories|7g carbohydrates|8g protiens|9g fat

Ingredients

- 1⁄3 cup oil of vegetables
- Corn tortillas, sliced into wedges
- 1⁄2 red onion, diced
- Garlic cloves, minced
- 1 (7 oz) el pato sauce (or 1 cup tomato sauce and a diced jalapeño)
- 1⁄2 teaspoon of salt
- 2-4 eggs

The optional toppings

- Cilantro, avocado, red onion sliced, cheese grated, fresh slices of lime

Directions

1. Heat the oil over high heat in a skillet. Place the tortilla triangles in a single layer once the oil is heated, and fry for several minutes till golden brown, tossing once. Remove and set aside to drain on a paper towel. For the remainder of the tortillas, repeat the process.
2. Reduce the heat to medium. Apply the remaining oil to the red onions and sauté for a couple of minutes before they start to soften. Add the garlic and sauté for around 30 seconds, then add to the skillet the tomato sauce, salt, and a handful of water. Simmer, and add the fried tortillas to the mix. Stir to coat.
3. Shift the tortillas to the outer edges of the skillet to cook the eggs to make a well in the center. You should scramble or cover the pan to encourage them to simply poach in the sauce. Drop the eggs into the sauce and cook them to your taste.
4. Serve with the toppings.

6. Sausage Sandwich with Honey Sriracha Sauce

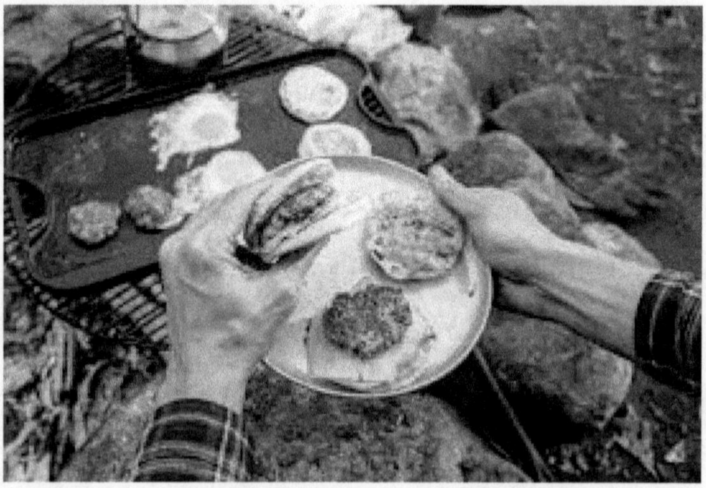

Serving: 6

Preparation time: 15 minutes

Nutritional Values: 600kcal calories|12g carbohydrates|19g protiens|35g fat

Ingredients

Sausage Patties

- 1 pound of ground pork
- Dried herbs, around 2 teaspoons: thyme, rosemary, sage, etc.
- 1 teaspoon of salt

Sriracha Honey Sauce

- 1/2 cup of honey
- Tablespoon of Sriracha

Assemble the Sandwich

- Eggs
- Slices of cheese
- Breakfast muffins / English muffins

Directions

1. **Prep the sausages:** In a broad bowl, combine the ground pork, herbs, and salt until
2. completely mixed. Morph into 6 patties of similar percentage, bearing in mind that when

cooking, they can shrink slightly.

3. **Prep the Sauce:** In a small bowl, mix the honey and Sriracha together and whisk together. Then set aside.
4. **Cook:** Over the campfire or stovetop, heat a griddle or skillet. Place the sausages on the surface until heated, then cook until browned for 2-3 minutes. Flip and cook until browned on the other hand for another 2-3 minutes. Meanwhile, as needed, cook the eggs and toast the English muffins.
5. **Organize & Serve:** Spread on the English muffins the Sriracha honey sauce, then layer with a sausage patty, egg, and cheese slice. Serve and enjoy.

7. Chickpea Breakfast Hash with Veggies

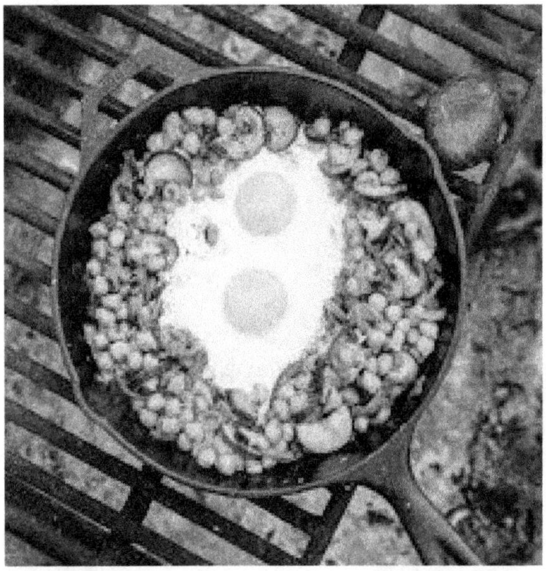

Serving: 2

Preparation time: 20 minutes

Nutritional values: 379kcal calories|12g carbohydrates|13g protiens|8g fat

Ingredients

- 1 tablespoon of oil
- 1 summer squash or zucchini, divided into half-moons of 1/2-inch
- 1 tiny red onion, divided into half-moons of 1/4-inch
- mini sweet peppers or 1 bell pepper, sliced into 1/4-inch slices

- 1 (15 oz.) chickpeas, drained Can
- 1/2 teaspoon of cumin
- 1/4 teaspoon coriander
- 1/8 teaspoon cinnamon
- About 1/2 teaspoon salt, and more to taste
- Eggs

Directions

1. On a medium-high flame, heat the oil in a skillet over the campfire or camp stove unless hot and glinting. Include the onions, peppers, and zucchini and sauté for around 5 minutes before it starts to soften. Incorporate the drained chickpeas and spices and simmer for around 10 minutes, until the vegetables and chickpeas are cooked and browned in portions.
2. To make a well in the center of the plate, transfer the vegetables & chickpeas to the sides of the skillet. If the bottom of the pan is looking dry, apply a little oil. In the well, break two eggs and cook them to your taste.
3. Remove the skillet from the flame and serve.

8. Banana Coconut French Toast

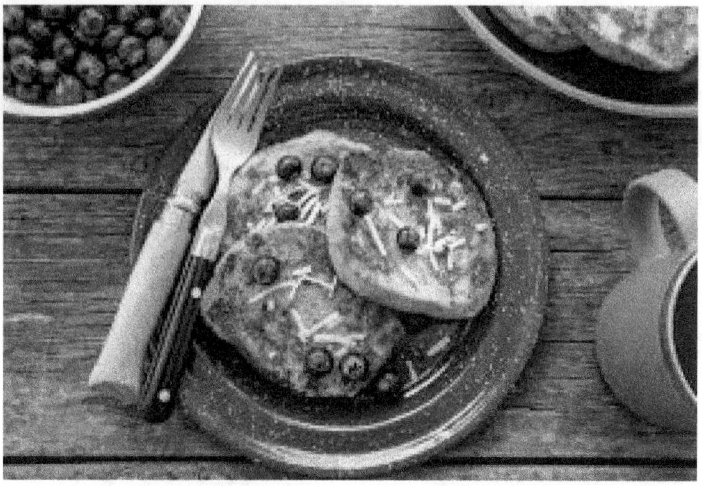

Serving: 4

Preparation time: 30 minutes

Nutritional values: 360kcal calories|8g carbohydrates|9g protiens|12g fat

Ingredients

- 1 lb. loaf of crusty French bread, sliced into 3/4-inch pieces
- 1 quite ripe banana
- 1 (14 oz.) of coconut milk Can
- 1 teaspoon of cinnamon ground
- 1 teaspoon extract of vanilla
- 1/2 tsp of salt
- Coconut oil

To serve

- Warmed Maple Syrup Substitute
- Fresh blueberries
- Shredded flakes of coconut

Directions

1. Mash the banana until it is soft in a bowl wide enough to fit a slice or two of bread. Incorporate the coconut milk, cinnamon, vanilla extract, and salt and whisk to blend. You want as smooth as possible for this batter.
2. Over medium heat, prepare a nonstick pan.
3. Dip a slice of bread into the batter and let it soak on each side for a couple of seconds. Let the excess runoff and then fry it on each side, around 3 minutes per side, in the skillet until golden and crispy.
4. Repeat with the rest of the bread, adding to the pan the coconut oil as required.
5. Enjoy with syrup, fresh blueberries, and shredded coconut. Serve and enjoy.

9. Huevos Rancheros Verdes

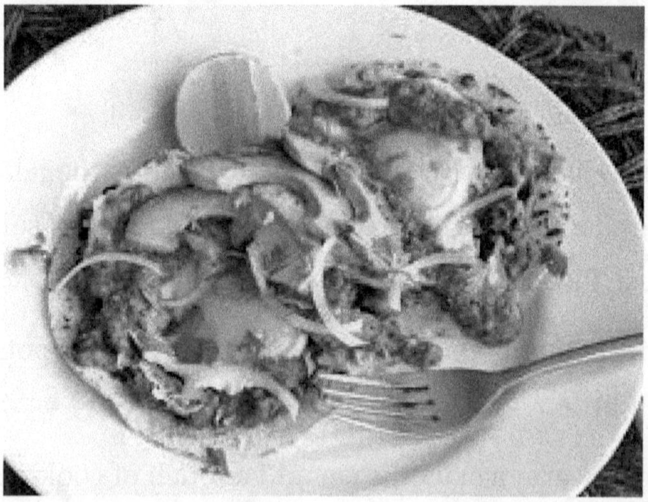

Serving: 2

Preparation time: 35 minutes

Nutritional values: 350kcal calories|10g carbohydrates|12g protiens|9g fat

Ingredients

- oz. jar of Verde salsa
- Eggs
- tortillas of corn
- Cooking Oil
- 1 avocado, sliced
- 1 lime, chopped into wedges
- Fresh cilantro
- 1 Oz. Pico de Gallo, (store-purchased, or see below recipe)

Fresh Pico de Gallo

- A handful of cherry tomatoes quartered or halved
- 1/4 minced white onion
- 1 jalapeno, de-seeded and chopped
- 1 lime, juiced

- 1/8 teaspoon salt
- Fresh cilantro, chopped

Directions

1. Make the Pico de Gallo: Halve or quarter the tomatoes, chop the jalapeno, de-seed and mince the onions, and cut the cilantro. Place the lime juice and a pinch of salt in a small cup. Set aside. (Note: You may also use Pico de Gallo obtained from the store!)
2. Set over medium-low heat and pour the salsa Verde into a small pot. Carry to a trickle and let it reduce and thicken a little.
3. Over medium-high heat, warm a skillet, then add a touch of cooking oil. In the pan, toast the tortillas until browned in patches, then set aside.
4. Reduce the heat to medium. If needed, add more oil to the pan (be generous).
5. Crack the eggs into the skillet. Cook until the eggs are ready to your taste, tilting the pan as appropriate to spread the oil across the sides equally.
6. Lay two tortillas on a plate to serve and place the eggs on top. Spillover the tops of the warmed salsa Verde, and top with Pico de Gallo, avocado, cilantro, a sprinkle of salt, and a lime squeeze.

10. Turmeric Tofu Scramble

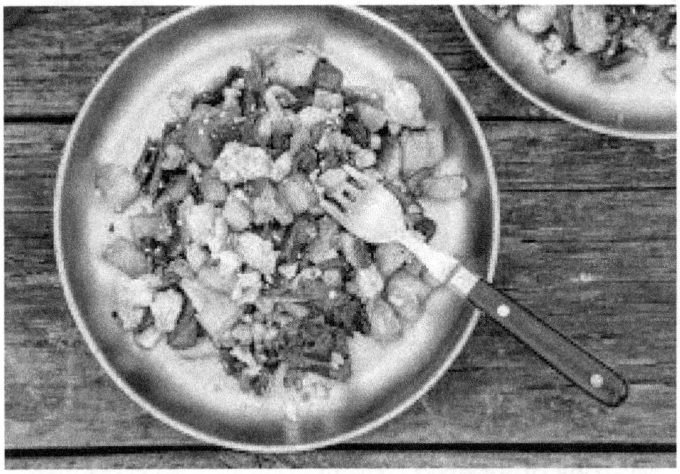

Serving: 2

Preparation time: 15 minutes

Nutritional values: 270kcal calories|16g carbohydrates|14g protiens|18g fat

Ingredients

- 2 tablespoons of oil
- Mini potatoes fingerlings
- Mushrooms
- 1 tiny shallot
- 2 cups of spinach
- Tofu around 5 oz, pat dry with a paper towel
- 1⁄4 teaspoon of turmeric
- 1 tablespoon of nutritional yeast
- 1⁄4 teaspoon of salt
- 1 pinch of black pepper

Directions

1. Cut the potatoes into 1⁄4" cubes. Cut the mushrooms in the quarter. Slice into half-moons the shallot.
2. Over medium heat, heat a tbsp of oil in a pan. When heated, add the potatoes and cook for around 7 minutes, until they start to soften and turn brown. Add the shallots and mushrooms and cook for three minutes, until the mushrooms start to brown and the shallots are tender. Shift to one of the pans' sides.
3. If required, add another tablespoon of oil. Crumble in the pan the tofu and toss with the oil. Dust the turmeric over the tofu and nutritional yeast, then sauté for 4 minutes.
4. Transfer the spinach to the pan, then swirl until simmered with the other components of the scramble.
5. Add salt & pepper to taste. Enjoy.

11. Coconut Chocolate Granola

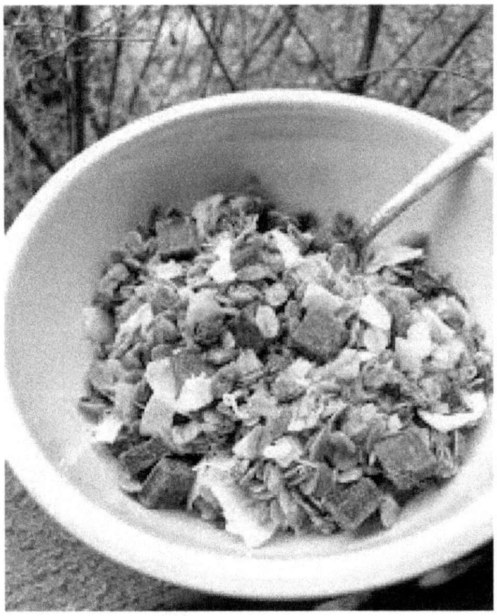

Serving: 4

Preparation time: 20 minutes

Nutritional values: 614kcal caloreis|53g carbohydrates|11g protiens|42g fat

Ingredients

- 1 cup of oats, rolled
- 1/2 cup of chopped nuts
- 1/4 cup of cacao powder
- 1/4 cup of maple syrup
- 2 tablespoons melted coconut oil
- 1 pinch of salt
- 1 cup of coconut flakes
- tbsp of powdered milk
- 1 oz of Freeze-dried raspberries or other freeze-dried fruit

Directions

1. Preheat the oven to 300F
2. Combine the oats, nuts, cacao powder, maple syrup, molten coconut oil, and salt in a wide bowl

until it is covered evenly.

3. Pour the mixture on a baking sheet lined with parchment paper in an even layer. Bake it for 15 minutes.
4. Remove from the oven the baking sheet, incorporate the coconut, and return for an extra 5 minutes to the oven.
5. Take the granola out of the oven and let it cool fully.
6. Divide the granola into 4 bags of zip tops. To each bag, add 1 tablespoon powdered milk and 1⁄4 oz of freeze-dried raspberries.

At the Camp

1. Add half a cup of water (hot or cold) to the bag at camp and blend. Enjoy your breakfast.

12. Blueberry Banana Pancakes

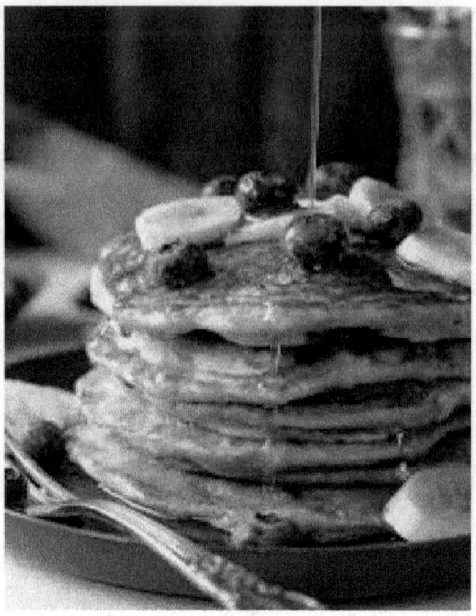

Serving: 6

Preparation time: 30 minutes

Nutritional values: 185kcal calories|17g carbohydrates|29g proteins|16g fat

Ingredients

- 1 cup of flour
- 1⁄3 cup milk powder + 1 cup water / 1 cup milk
- teaspoons sugar

- 1 teaspoon baking powder roughly
- 1⁄4 teaspoon of salt
- 1 egg
- 1 banana, split into 1/4 "inch chunks."
- 1/2 cup of blueberries
- teaspoons of ghee or butter

Serving

- Maple syrup, butter, jam or creamed honey

Directions

1. In a bowl, blend the flour, powdered milk, baking powder and salt (this can be done in advance at home and placed in a resealable bag or container). Add the dry ingredients to the water and egg. Use a fork to whisk the ingredients to mix, making sure not to mix too much (some little lumps in the batter are okay),
2. Heat a skillet over medium-low heat over your campfire or camp stove. Add a teaspoon of ghee to the skillet and move to coat the pan. Add 1⁄3 cup of the pancake batter into the middle of the skillet and place it on top of each of the banana slices and blueberries. Cook for a couple of minutes before the top starts to bubble, and the sides are set (about 2-3 minutes). Turn the pancake and use a spatula.
3. Repeat with the rest of the batter and, if needed, apply 1 teaspoon of ghee to the pan for each pancake.
4. Stack the pancakes to eat and line with maple syrup, jam, butter, or honey. Eat and enjoy.

13. Johnny Apple Seed Oatmeal

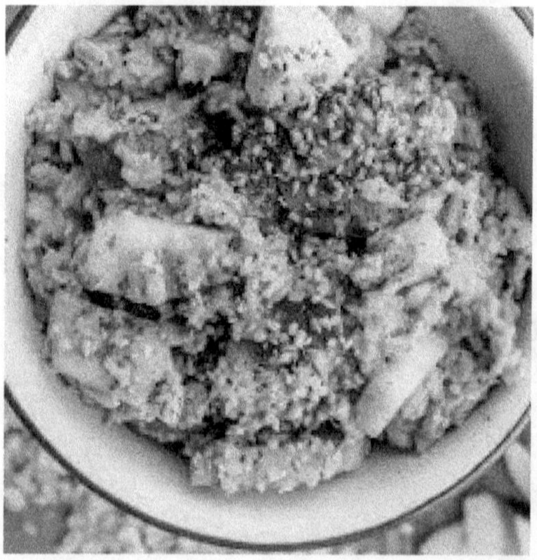

Serving: 2

Preparation time: 12 minutes

Nutritional values: 300kcal calories| 10g carbohydrates| 9g proteins|6g fat

Ingredients

- Cups of water
- A pinch of salt
- 1 cup of rolled oats
- 1 medium-sized apple, sliced into 1/2 pieces
- 1/2 tsp of grounded cinnamon
- 1/4 tsp of grounded nutmeg
- 1/4 tsp of grounded cloves
- 1/4 teaspoon of allspice
- 1-2 tbsp. of hemp, chia seeds or flax
- 2 tbsp of maple syrup

Direction

1. In a medium pot, heat the salt and water until it begins to boil.
2. Integrate the oats, boil for around 10 min, or stir periodically till the oats are soft.

3. Add the apple, seasonings, and maple syrup midway through the cooking process.

14. Shakshuka

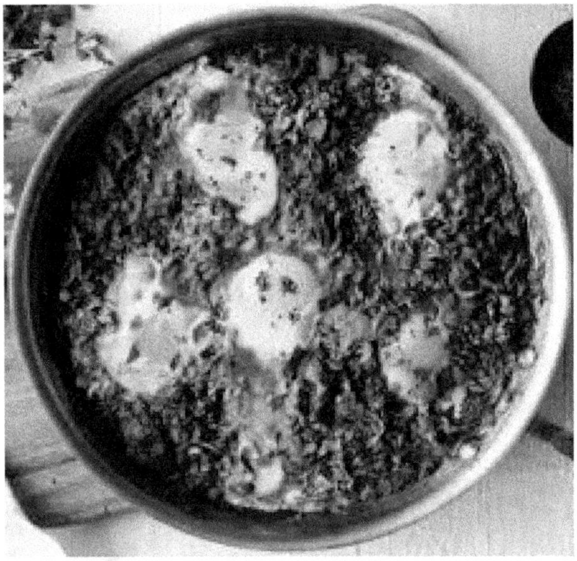

Serving: 2

Preparation time: 25 minutes

Nutritional values: 276kcal calories|23g carbohydrates|12g proteins|16g fat

Ingredients

- 1 tbsp of olive oil
- 1 red seeded and diced bell pepper
- 1 seeded and sliced poblano peppers,
- 1 tiny onion, chopped
- 1 tsp. of garlic cloves, minced
- 1 tsp. of paprika
- 1 tsp of cumin
- 14 oz of diced canned tomatoes
- 2 eggs
- 1/4 cup of feta cheese
- Parsley, minced

- Pepper and salt

Directions

1. On medium heat, add the oil to your pan. Once the poblano and red bell peppers and onions are hot, swirl to coat, and cook for 5 minutes or until brown, stirring if necessary. Add the garlic, paprika and cumin and simmer for around 30 seconds until it is fragrant.
2. Put in the tomatoes and their juices. To enable the mixture to stiffen, reduce the heat and cook for 10 minutes.
3. In the sauce, smash the eggs, spaced them uniformly apart. Cover until the whites are set, and the yolk is to your desired consistency, 5-7 minutes, and allow the eggs to cook. To enable them to cook thoroughly, you may spoon the sauce over the top as desired.
4. Season it to taste. Serve right away with feta cheese, minced parsley and a few crusty bread slices.

15. Apple and Sweet Potato Hash

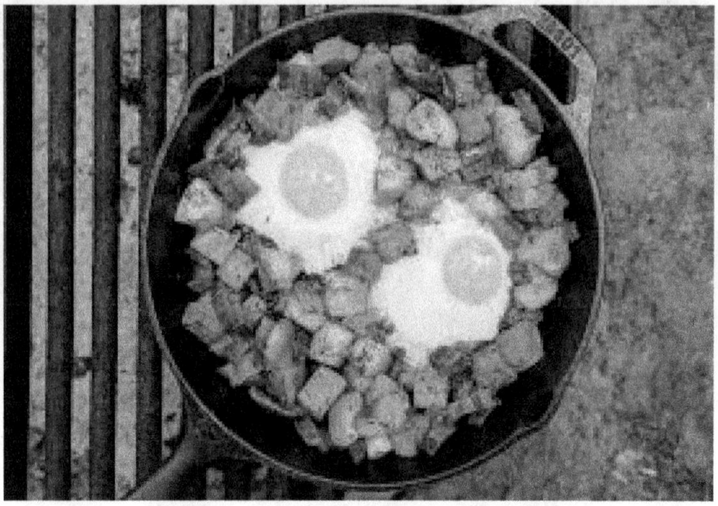

Serving: 2

Preparation time: 20 minutes

Nutritional values: 462k calories|14g carbohydrates|14g proteins|38g fat

Ingredients

- Slices of thick-cut bacon (the Black Forest, if you can reach it)
- 1 sweet medium potato (skinned if preferred)

- 1 granny smith apple
- 1 tsp of thyme
- 1 tbsp of butter (optional)
- 2 eggs

Directions

1. In 1/2 to 1-inch chunks, cut the sweet potato and apple.
2. In a pan, add the bacon. Turn on a medium burner. Fry the bacon so that it just begins to crisp on the rim, then turn and cook for an extra minute or so. Remove and put on a plate that is lined with paper towels and set aside.
3. Put in the skillet the sweet potato, apple, and a bit of salt, and sauté for around 15 minutes until tender. Chop the bacon in the meantime. Transfer the bacon to the skillet and scatter with the thyme when the sweet potato and apples are almost done. Taste and, if needed, add salt.
4. Place the hash around to build two wells in order to cook the eggs. You should apply a bit of butter to each well if the skillet has dried out, to let the eggs cook and avoid sticking. In each well, break an egg and cook to your taste.
5. Immediately serve & enjoy your breakfast.

16. Grilled Halloumi Breakfast Sandwich

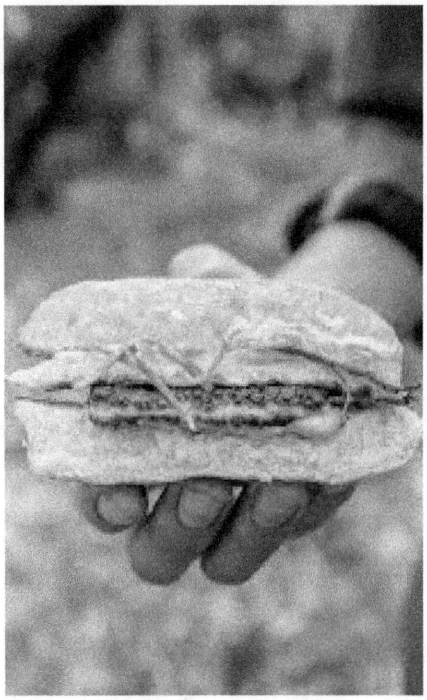

Serving: 1

Preparation time: 20 minutes

Nutritional values: 651kcal calories|17g carbohydrates| 12g proteins|23g fat

Ingredients

- 1 large sweet Hawaiian roll (if you can manage them, use the sandwich buns)
- 1 tablespoon of butter or oil, divided,
- Halloumi cheese 2 oz, sliced
- 1 egg
- 1-2 tbsp. of mayo
- 1 tablespoon of Sriracha, (more or less according to your choice for heat)
- 1 scallion, julienned or diced
- Salt + pepper, for flavor

Directions

1. Either in your pan or on a grill, toast the sandwich buns. And set aside.
2. Over medium-high heat, melt half the butter or oil in your skillet. Add the cheese until melted. Fry in spots on either side until golden brown, approximately 3-4 minutes on either side. And set aside. If you've got one going, this move may also be achieved on a barbecue. Skip the butter/oil in that scenario and put the cheese directly on the grill.
3. Over medium heat, add butter or oil. Crack the egg into the pan until it is melted. Totally optional step: You should use a fork to blend the yolk a little until the whites begin to set so that it gets spread a little around the egg, so there will be yolk in every bit. Cook the egg for around 4 minutes or until it's cooked to the perfect degree of doneness.
4. Prepare the spicy mayo when the egg is cooking. Mix the mayo and the Sriracha together in a tiny bowl (or in a measuring cup).
5. To combine, on each cut surface of the buns, distribute the spicy mayo. Layer to taste with the grilled halloumi, egg, scallions, and salt & pepper.

17. Asparagus Pancetta Skillet Hash

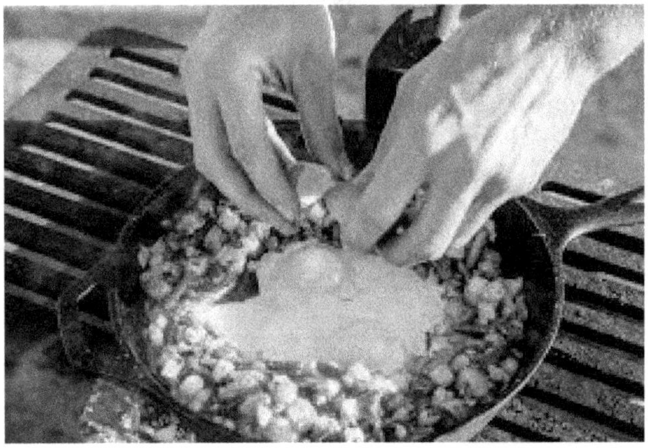

Serving: 2

Preparation time: 25 minutes

Nutritional values: 380kcal calories|8g carbohydrates|13g proteins|21g fat

Ingredients

- 1 tablespoon of oil
- 1 medium potato, peeled, sliced into 1/4-inch dice if needed
- 1 asparagus bunch, sliced into 1-inch fragments
- 3-4 oz. pancetta, diced (we use Trader Joe's pre-diced pancetta)
- 1 garlic clove, minced
- 1/4 teaspoon sea salt and more to taste
- 2-3 eggs

Directions

1. **Cook the potatoes:** Heat the oil on your stovetop or on a grill over your campfire in a cast-iron skillet over moderate heat. Add the potatoes in an even layer until the oil is hot. Cook for around 8 minutes, rotating periodically until the potatoes begin to turn crispy so that both sides have a chance to brown.
2. **Cook the asparagus & pancetta:** Add to your skillet the asparagus, pancetta, garlic, and sea salt. For an additional 8-10 minutes, proceed to cook until the pancetta is golden and the asparagus is heated through and moist.
3. **Fry the eggs:** To make a well in the center of the skillet, move the hash to the side. Break the

eggs into the well and prepare them for the perfect doneness (to produce a solid white and a runny yolk, close the skillet and cook for 3 minutes).

4. **Serve:** Serve directly, either in a shared skillet or split into two pans.

18. Chorizo and Sweet Potato Hash

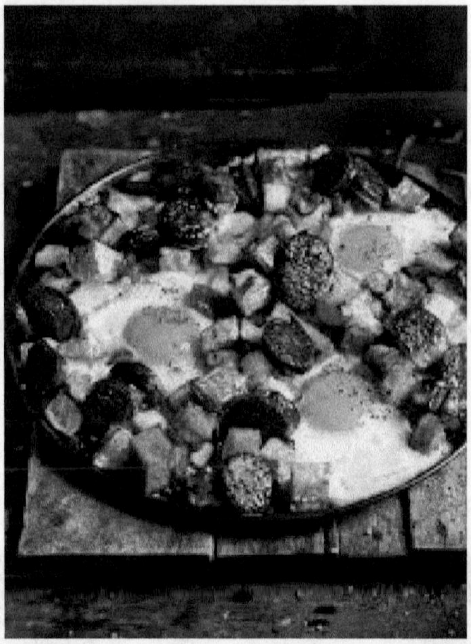

Serving: 2

Preparation time: 20 minutes

Nutritional values: 267kcal calories|4g carbohydrates|12g proteins|22g fat

Ingredients

- 1 sweet potato medium-size, peeled if wanted
- Green onions
- 1 tablespoon of oil
- 2 oz crumbly chorizo or soyrizo
- 1 teaspoon of maple syrup
- 1/8 tsp of cinnamon
- 2 eggs
- Salt to flavor

Directions

1. Slice the sweet potato into 1/4-1/2-inch cubes and cut the green onions (green + light green sections) finely.
2. Heat oil over medium-high heat in a skillet. Add the sweet potato until the oil glints. Shake to coat, then simmer for 5 minutes, stirring periodically, until tender.
3. Stir in the green onions and simmer for an extra 5 minutes.
4. Add the chorizo until the potatoes are soft. Cook for 2 minutes or until thoroughly cooked. Add the cinnamon and maple syrup and season with salt if desired. Stir to mix.
5. In the hash, make two wells and break an egg into each. Then cook the eggs to your taste. To make sunny side up eggs, cover the skillet with a lid for around 2 minutes.
6. Enjoy the breakfast.

19. Camping Croissant Sandwich

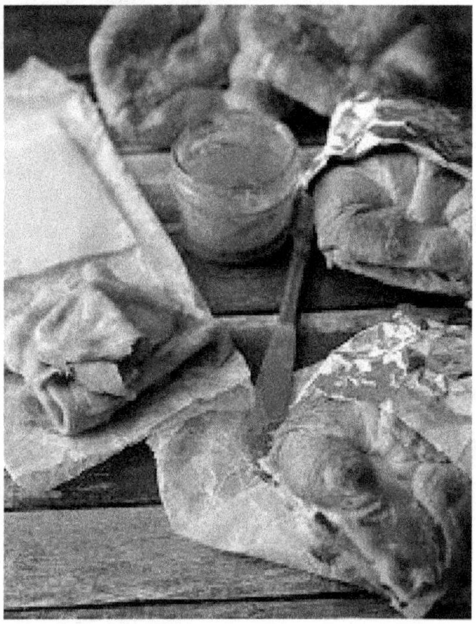

Serving: 4

Preparation time: 20 minutes

Nutritional values: 314kcal calories|13g carbohydrates|9g proteins|12g fat

Ingredients

- 4 eggs of large size

- 4 slices of cheese, your choice in flavor
- 2-3 slices of chosen Canadian bacon or meat, such as cooked bacon, ham or sausage
- 4 croissants, or the option of bread
- 4 tablespoons of butter
- Portable grill or fire grill

Directions

At the campsite

1. Cut your croissants and spread them with the butter. Then set aside.
2. On a preheated cooking surface, crack the eggs. Season with salt and pepper to taste. Cook for 1-2 minutes and flip.
3. On each egg, put one slice of cheese and enable it to melt when it completes cooking on the second side.
4. Place the meat of your preference on the grill to cook it up. To toast, put the sliced croissants cut side, down.
5. Create and serve your sandwich.

Make ahead

Cooking on a stovetop, observe the following directions.

1. On a square of foil, place the stacked sandwiches. Wrap and freeze securely.
2. At the campsite: On hot coals or a grill, heat the sandwiches until warm.
3. Serve and enjoy

3.2 Lunch and Dinner Recipes

1. Campfire Nachos

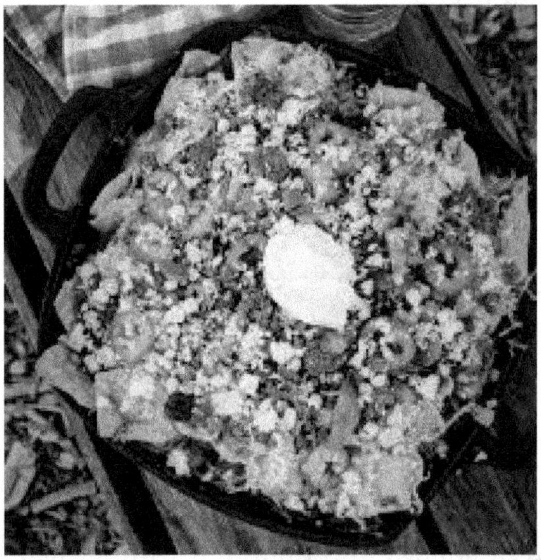

Serving: 2

Preparation time: 15 minutes

Nutritional values: 987kcal calories|125g carbohydrates|213g proteins|345g fat

Ingredients

- 1 tablespoon of a neutral flavor
- 1⁄2 pound of tortilla chips
- 1 (7.75 oz.) Can of El Pato hot tomato sauce, or equal
- 1 cup shredded Mexican cheese mix
- 1 (14.5 oz.) Can of black beans, washed
- 1 large, diced avocado
- 4-5 green, sliced onions
- A handful of fresh, chopped cilantro
- 1 small lime, sliced into wedges

Directions

1. To avoid the nachos from sticking, gently grease the bottom of a broad Dutch oven.

2. Spread 1⁄3 of the chips thinly into the Dutch oven for the first layer, covered with 1⁄4 of a Can of El Pato, 1⁄4 of black beans, 1⁄4 of a cup of cheese, and a bunch of avocados, green onions, and cilantro. For the second layer, repeat.
3. Using the remaining 1⁄3 part of chips, 1⁄2 Can El Pato, 1⁄2 Can of black beans, 1⁄2 cup cheese, and the remainder avocado, onion, and cilantro for the third and final layer.
4. Cover the Dutch oven and put it over your campfire on a metal grill for around 10 minutes before the cheese is melted. With the lime wedges, serve and enjoy.

2. Tzatziki Chicken Skewers

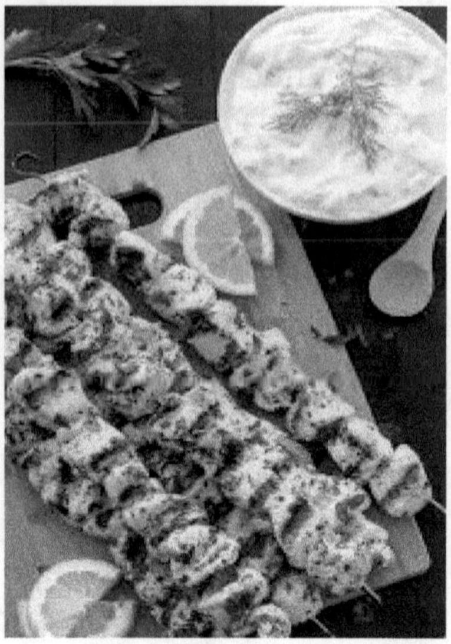

Serving: 2

Preparation time: 40 minutes

Nutritional values: 527kcal calories|13g carbohydrates|52g proteins|30g fat

Ingredients

- 2 tbsps. of oil, should be of olive
- 1 juiced lemon
- 1 tbsp of dry oregano
- 1/2 tsp powder of garlic
- 1/2 tsp of salt
- boneless thighs of skinless chicken, divided into 1.'

- 1 tiny zucchini, cut into moons of 1/4'
- 1 onion, diced
- 14 tomatoes of cherry
- Half cup tzatziki can be used as the store-purchased or recipe prepared as follows.

For Tzatziki Sauce

- Half cup of Greek yogurt
- 1/4 of cucumber, seeds should be separated & finely chopped
- 1 tablespoon of fresh mint, chopped
- 2 pieces of garlic, finely minced, finely minced
- 1/4 tsp of salt

Directions

1. Put the oil, lemon juice, garlic powder, oregano and a pinch of salt together in a bowl. To coat, apply and throw the chicken. Set aside for 30 minutes (up to 2 hours) to marinate, stirring intermittently.
2. To make Tzatziki (it is possible to make it before):
3. Blotting with a towel absorbs extra dampness from the sliced cucumber. In a small bowl, put the cucumber, yogurt, garlic, mint and salt, and blend to combine.
4. If finished ahead of time, wrap & preserve in the cooler.
5. For grilling, arrange a grate or a campfire.
6. Thread into skewers the chicken and veggies.
7. Put the skewers on the grill grate and cook as the grill is ready, rotating every few moments so that both sides cook equally. It will take the chicken 4-5 minutes to cook on either side, and it will take between 9-12 minutes for the vegetables.
8. Remove the skewers. For dipping, serve with tzatziki. Enjoy.

3. Shrimp Boil Foiled Packets

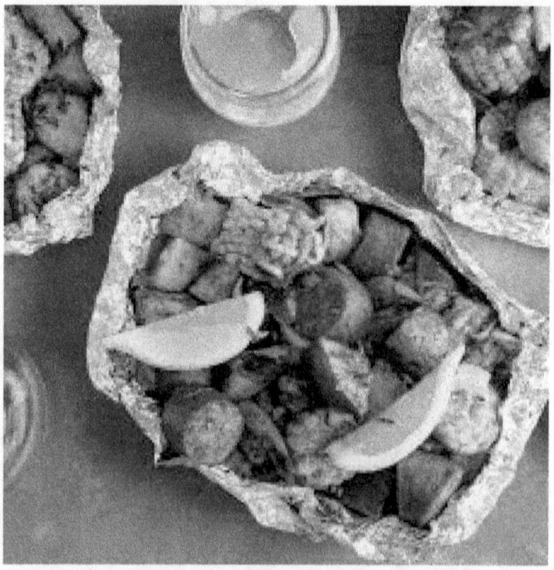

Serving: 2

Preparation time: 15 minutes

Nutritional values: 520kcal calories|23g carbohydrates|31g proteins|34g fat

Ingredients

- 1 ear of corn, sliced into eight pieces
- 1 medium zucchini, thickly sliced
- 4 teaspoons minced garlic
- 1/2 lb. shrimp, uncooked
- Andouille
- 1 teaspoon, Old Bay Seasoning
- 1 teaspoon of Cajun seasoning
- 1-2 of butter
- Chopped fresh parsley

Directions

1. For each packet, tear an 18 "strip of heavy-duty foil, along with a 16" piece of parchment paper for each. Layer the paper of parchment on top of the foil.
2. Between the two sheets of foil distribute the zucchini, corn, shrimp, minced garlic, spices, and

butter.

3. Bring one of the short sides of the foil to reach the other to shape the packets, then crimp along all the edges to secure.
4. Cook the packets for 8 minutes on a grill (or the grill pit over your campfire), tossing them frequently.
5. Take it off the grill and let it cool slightly. Carefully open the packets-they would be full of hot steam. Top and cherish with fresh parsley.

4. Chickpea Curry with Coconut Milk

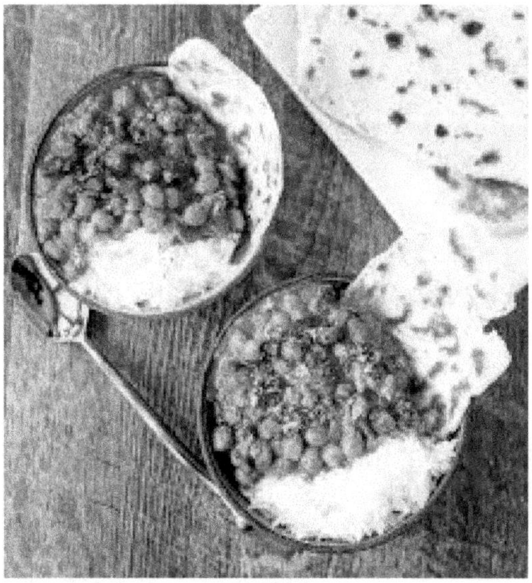

Serving: 4

Preparation time: 25 minutes

Nutritional values: 358kcal calories|39g carbohydrates|9g proteins|23g fat

Ingredients

- 1 tablespoon of oil or ghee
- 1 tiny onion, diced
- 1 tbsp of Garam Masala
- 1 tsp of cinnamon
- 1 tsp of ginger field
- 1 teaspoon of turmeric from the ground

- 1⁄4 cayenne pepper, optional; omit for milder heat
- 1 teaspoon of salt
- 1 tbsp tomato paste
- 1 (14 oz.) Can of coconut milk
- 1 (14 oz.) chickpeas, drained Can
- 1 lime, chopped into wedges
- Cilantro handful, sliced
- 1⁄4 cup of yogurt, optional, free from plain dairy or Greek

Directions

1. On medium heat, heat the oil or ghee in a pan and add the onions, stir-frying until crispy but not browning.
2. Add the garam masala, turmeric, ground ginger, cinnamon, then cayenne, and toast the spices momentarily to make them fragrant.
3. Add the tomato paste, coconut milk, and salt. Stir until the tomato paste in the coconut milk is fully mixed, then incorporate the chickpeas.
4. Cook over medium to medium-low heat, stirring regularly, for 10 to 15 minutes, until the sauce thickens to your taste.
5. Meanwhile, prepare the sides.
6. With a squeeze of lime, a dollop of yogurt (optional), serve the chickpea curry and garnish it with plenty of cilantro.

5. Chicken Pad Thai

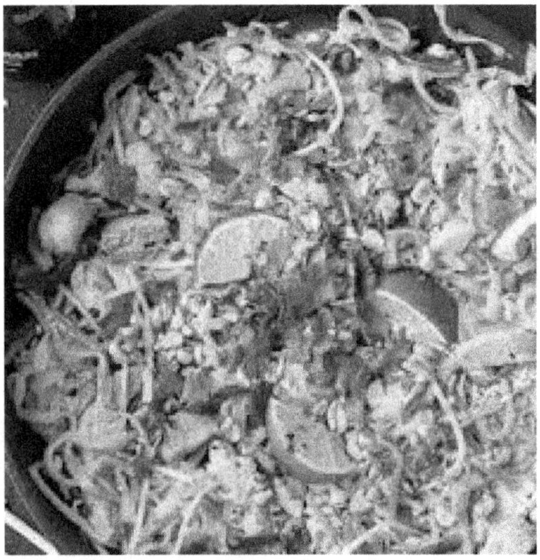

Serving: 2

Preparation time: 20 minutes

Nutritional values: 571kcal calories|31g carbohydrates|42g proteins|33g fat

Ingredients

- 7 oz Thai Pad Noodles
- 1 tbsp. of sesame oil
- 1 large breast of chicken, sliced into cubes
- 1 tiny onion, diced
- 1⁄4 teaspoon of salt
- 2-3 eggs, beaten
- 2⁄3 cup Pad Thai sauce, store-bought, or see the following recipe
- 1⁄2 cup of green onions diced
- 1⁄2 cup chopped cilantro
- 1⁄4 cup of minced peanuts

Thai Pad Sauce

- 2 tbsp of soy sauce
- 2 tbsp rice vinegar

- 2 tbsp of lime juice
- 2 tbsp brown sugar
- 1 tablespoon of chili-garlic or Sriracha Sauce
- 1 tablespoon fish sauce

Directions

1. Take a pan to boil water. Turn off the heat once the water is boiling and drench the noodles for 8-10 minutes. When they are soft but "al dente," noodles are done.
2. Meanwhile, heat 2 tbsp of sesame oil (or, if that's what you have, standard vegetable oil) in a medium saucepan. Add the chicken, onions, and salt until it is hot. Sauté until the chicken is completely cooked and the onions tend to brown.
3. Shift the chicken to one side of the pan, reduce the heat, then add the eggs to the skillet and whisk to scramble frequently.
4. Use tongs to pick the noodles out of their soaking water after the noodles are done, the chicken is cooked completely, and the eggs are scrambled. To the skillet, transfer the noodles and then mix in the Pad Thai sauce. To coat the noodles, stir the skillet.
5. Place green onions, fresh coriander, and chopped peanuts on top. Enjoy!

Optional Move at Home (if you don't want Pad Thai sauce bought from the store)

1. In a small, sealable jar or container, mix all the sauce ingredients and shake to combine. Pack it in a cooler.

6. Dutch Oven Mac and Cheese

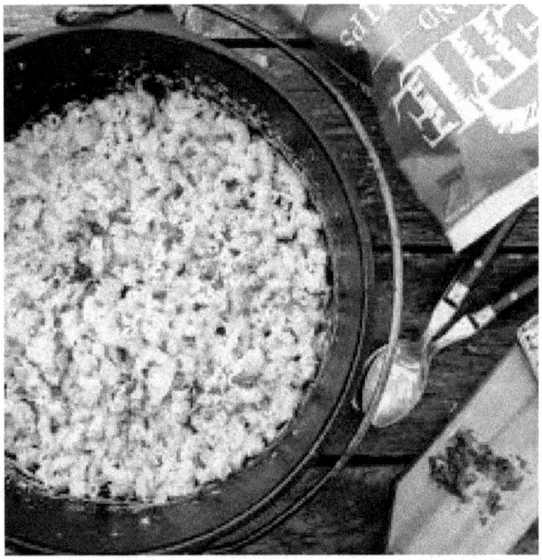

Serving: 4

Preparation time: 15 minutes

Nutritional values: 922kcal calories|123g carbohydrates|213g proteins|315g fat

Ingredients

- 2 cups of elbow macaroni
- 4 cups of water
- 2 tablespoons of butter
- 1⁄4 teaspoon of salt
- 2-3 cups shredded cheddar cheese
- 1-2 tbsp mustard
- 1/4 teaspoon garlic powder
- 2-3 Oz. bag of kettle brand jalapeño chips

Directions

1. Make your coals or campfire ready.
2. To a 4-qt Dutch oven, add the macaroni, water, butter, and salt. Cover and put a tiny bed of coals or embers on top of it. Place the top of the Dutch oven with 10-15 coals. Cook for about 10 minutes until most (but not all) of the liquid has been drained, and the pasta is soft.

3. Remove the Dutch oven from the campfire very carefully and put the cover aside.
4. Stir in the shredded cheese, mustard and garlic powder and, if necessary, add more salt.
5. Serve in bowls or on a tray, and top with Kettle Brand chips of crushed jalapeño. Enjoy.

7. One-Pot Pasta Primavera

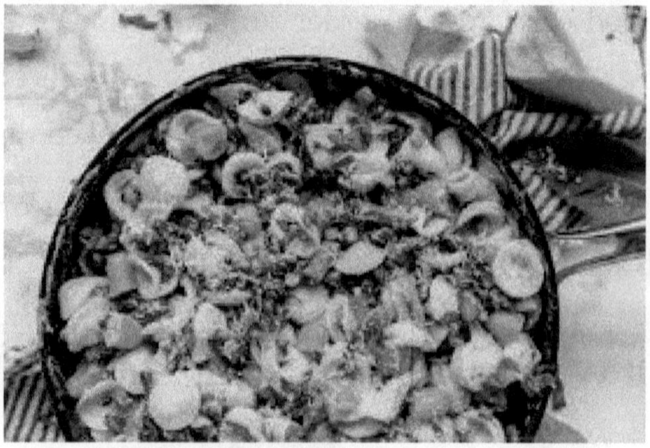

Serving: 2

Preparation time: 25 minutes

Nutritional values: 394kcal calories|51g carbohydrates|15g proteins|14g fat

Ingredients

- 1 zucchini
- 1 yellow summer squash
- 4 oz. Cherry Tomatoes
- cloves of garlic
- 1 tablespoon of oil
- 4 oz. Pasta
- 1 teaspoon of salt
- 2 oz. goat cheese
- Lemon juice, optional

Directions

1. Cut the squash and zucchini into 1⁄4-inch slices. Cut half of the cherry tomatoes. Then mince

the garlic.

2. In a high-sided skillet, heat the oil. When heated, add the vegetables and sauté for around 8 minutes until the squash is tender. Remove and set aside the vegetables from the skillet.
3. To the skillet, transfer the pasta, salt, and enough water to coat the pasta. Bring the water over medium heat to a boil and cook until the pasta is soft, around 10 minutes (depending on the pasta you use, this period can vary). In order to maintain even cooking, make sure to stir constantly. You should always add a little more of the water boils off until the pasta is tender. Remove the skillet from the heat as soon as the pasta has cooked through.
4. To coat the pasta, stir in the goat's cheese. Back to the skillet, incorporate the vegetables and stir to coat. Finish with a lemon squeeze, eat & enjoy.

8. Campfire Foil Wrapped Baked Sweet Potato Plus Chili

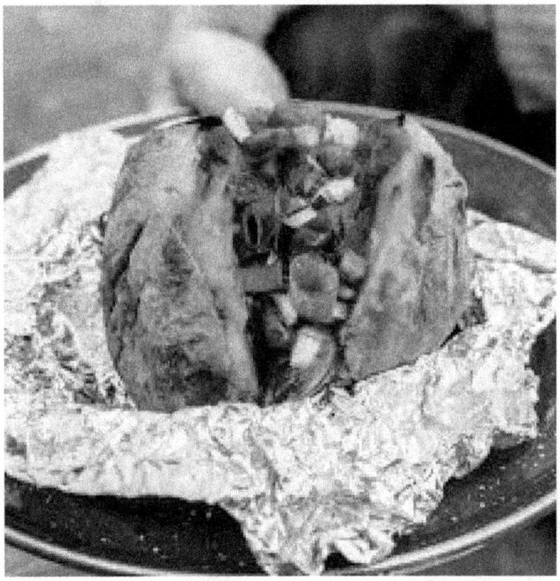

Serving: 4

Preparation time: 35 minutes

Nutritional values: 317kcal calories|9g carbohydrates|12g proteins|17g fat

Ingredients

- 4 medium sweet potatoes
- 1 onion, diced
- 1 tablespoon of olive oil

- 15 oz. Can of Kidney beans, drained
- 1 oz. tomato paste Can
- ½ Can of beer
- 1 tablespoon of chili powder
- ½ tbsp of cumin
- ½ teaspoon of salt
- Additional optional toppings contain green onions, cheese, avocado, etc.

Directions

1. Cover the heavy-duty foil in each of the sweet potatoes and nestle them in the campfire's embers. To ensure they cook uniformly, turn them each so often.
2. Make the chili when the potatoes are cooking. Heat the oil in the pot over medium heat. Add 3/4 of the diced onions until heated (reserve the remaining for topping) and sauté for a couple of minutes till they start to soften. Beans, tomato paste, beer (or other liquid, such as broth), and spices should be included. To mix, stir well. Steam for 15-20 minutes.
3. Regain from the fire once the potatoes are soft and cooked through (approximately 30 minutes max, give or take a bit based on their size). Unwrap the foil cautiously. To carve a slit into the potato, use a knife and top it with the chili, onions, and whatever else you have on hand. Enjoy.

9. African Sweet Potato and Peanut Stew

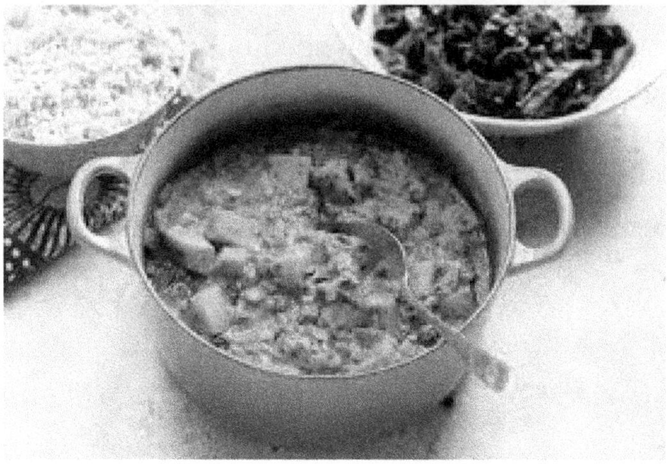

Serving: 4

Preparation time: 35 minutes

Nutritional values: 334kcal calories|9g carbohydrates|12g proteins|8g fat

Ingredients

- 1 tablespoon of oil
- 1 small, diced onion (to yield 1 1/2 cups)
- garlic cloves, minced (about 1 tablespoon)
- 1 medium sweet potato, diced into cubes of 1/4 inch (to provide 2 cups)
- 2-3 cups of broth
- 14 oz., tomatoes Can, diced
- 1/4 cup of peanut butter
- 2 teaspoons New Mexico chili powder
- 1 teaspoon of salt
- 14 oz. Can of chickpeas, processed
- 2 cups of Tuscan kale, scraped and chopped

Directions

1. Heat the oil over a moderate flame in a Dutch oven. Add the onion and sauté for about 5 minutes, until the onion is crispy and starts to brown in places. Add the garlic and sauté for around 1 minute until it is fragrant.
2. Include the sweet potato, broth, tomatoes & their juices, chili powder, peanut butter, and salt. To confirm that the peanut butter is fully blended in, whisk well, so there are no clumps left. Simmer, uncovered, or until the sweet potatoes are soft, for around 15-20 minutes.
3. Add the chickpeas and the kale to the Dutch oven once the sweet potatoes are tender. Stir to mix and cook until the chickpeas are warm and the kale wilts.

10. Cheesy Asparagus One Pot Orzo

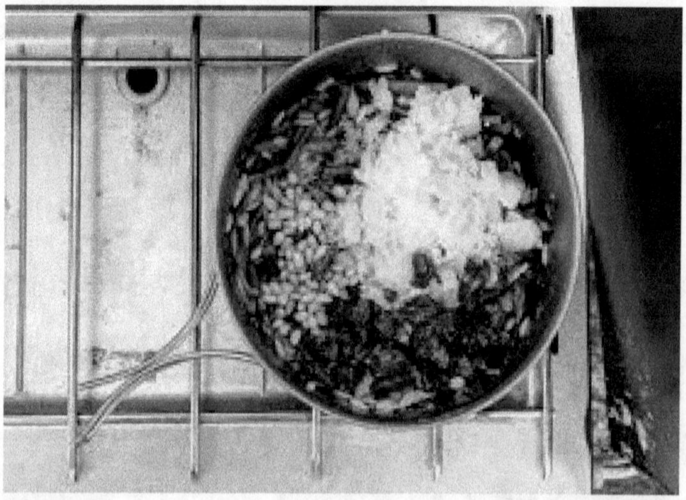

Serving: 2

Preparation time: 15 minutes

Nutritional values: 523kcal calories|70g carbohydrates|22g proteins|18g fat

Ingredients

- 1/2 lb. Asparagus
- 2 cups of water
- 1 cup of orzo
- 1/2 tablespoon olive oil
- 1/2 teaspoon of dry thyme
- 1/2 teaspoon basil dried
- 1/2 teaspoon garlic powder
- 1/2 tsp of salt
- 1/4 teaspoon flakes of red pepper
- 1/2 cup shredded cheese (you can use Trader Joe's 4 Cheese Mix, parmesan, asiago, or any blend)
- 1/4 cup of tomatoes sun-dried, chopped tbsp, pine nuts

Directions

1. Cut the rough ends of the asparagus off and discard them, and then slice the asparagus into 1-

inch bits.

2. In a bowl, add the asparagus, water, orzo, oil and all of the spices. Bring to a low simmer (this took 4 1/2 minutes) and simmer until the orzo is soft for an additional 5 minutes.
3. Add the cheese, sun-dried tomatoes, and pine nuts and turn the heat down. Stir until you've melted the cheese.
4. Remove from the heat, season with salt and pepper to taste, and enjoy.

11. Cilantro Lime Grilled Chicken Tacos

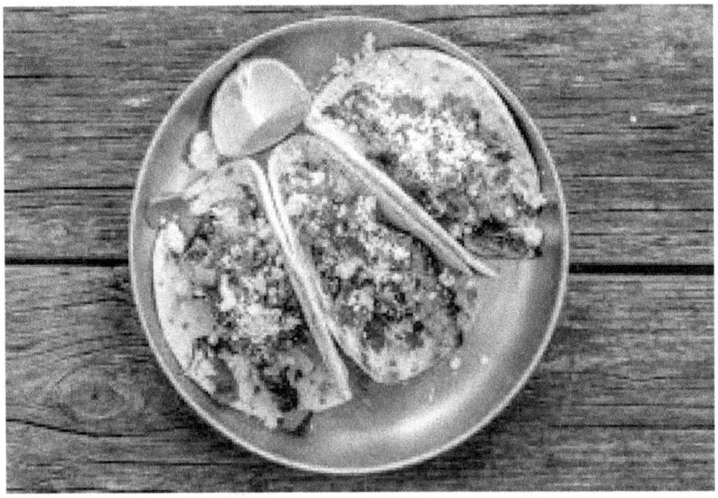

Serving: 4

Preparation time: 1 hour

Nutritional values: 275kcal calories|24g carbohydrates|21g proteins|11g fat

Ingredients

The marinade of Cilantro Lime

- 4 boneless skinless thighs of chicken, around 1 pound
- 1 tbsp. chopped cilantro
- limes, juice + zest
- 1 teaspoon of salt
- 1 teaspoon of chili powder
- 1 teaspoon of cumin
- 1⁄2 teaspoon garlic powder

- 1/2 teaspoon ground coriander
- 1 tablespoon of oil

For Assembling Taco

- Tortillas
- Pico de Gallo
- Cheese
- Cilantro

Directions

1. Start preparing the marinade: In a small bowl, blend together the oil, lime juice + zest, cilantro, and spices (this can be prepared at home). Place the chicken in a sealable container or Tupperware and spill over the marinade, shake to assure that the chicken is uniformly coated. Marinate for at least 30 minutes or up to 2 hours (an hour is better).
2. For grilling, set a grill or a campfire.
3. From the marinade, remove the chicken and put it on the grill. Cook until the inner temperature reaches 165F, changing as required to ensure even cooking (on each side for approximately 5-8 minutes). Remove from the heat and cut into sections that are bite-sized.
4. Layer Pico de Gallo, cheese, chicken and fresh cilantro onto tortillas to stack the tacos (warmed over the grill if you like) and enjoy them.

12. Pineapple Chicken Kabobs

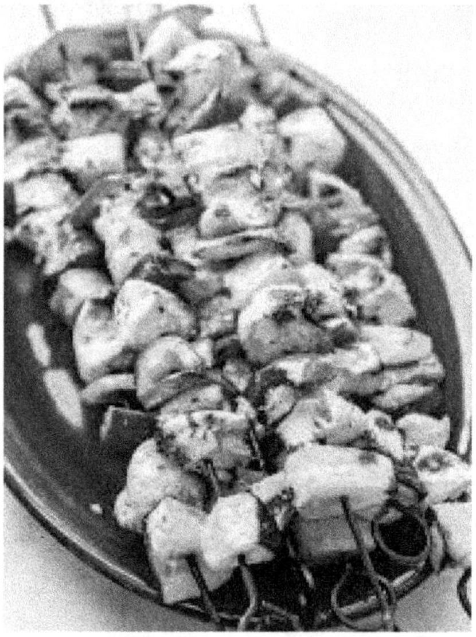

Serving: 4

Preparation time: 1 hour 20 minutes

Nutritional values: 275kcal calories|8g carbohydrates|11g proteins|22g fat

Ingredients

For the marinade

- 1⁄4 cup of olive oil
- 1⁄2 cup chopped cilantro
- 1 tablespoon of honey
- 2-3 teaspoons of minced ginger note: Trader Joe's stocks a great ginger paste for this.
- 1 lime, juiced
- 1 teaspoon of salt

For the skewers

- Chicken around 1⁄2 lb., boneless, skinless thighs fit best, sliced into pieces of 1 inch.
- 1 red medium onion, cut into 1-inch pieces
- Pineapple wedges, sliced into cubes of one inch

Directions

1. Combine the marinade components in a deep bowl or in a Ziplock bag.
2. Apply the marinade to the chicken and mix to coat it. Cover or close the container and allow to marinate for up to 24 hours or for at least an hour. If it takes more than an hour for you to marinate, put it back in your cooler.
3. Heat up your grill or get your campfire going in the meantime.
4. By stapling the chicken and vegetables onto the skewers make the kabobs. Brush it with some oil.
5. Grill the kabobs over medium-high to high flame, flipping them frequently so that they cook uniformly until the chicken is cooked through.
6. Take it out of the grill and enjoy.

13. Pie Iron Pizza Pockets

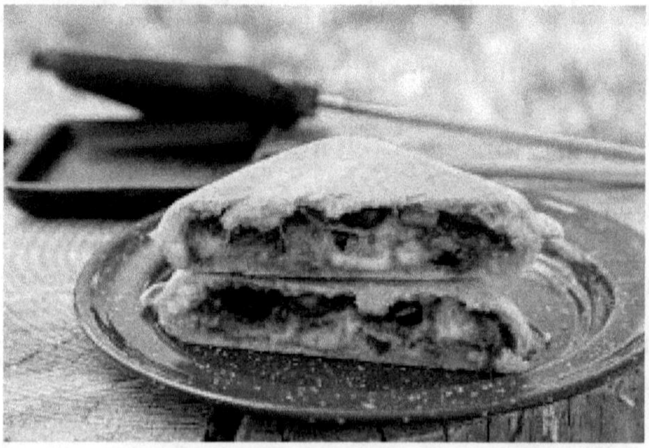

Serving: 4

Preparation time: 45 minutes

Nutritional values: 550kcal calories|67g carbohydrates|18g proteins|23g fat

Ingredients

Dough for Pizza

- 2&3⁄4 cups all-purpose flour
- 1 packet of yeast rapid rise
- 2 teaspoons of salt
- 1 cup of hot water
- 1 tbsp. of olive oil

The Fillings

- 1⁄2 cup of pizza sauce
- 1 cup of low-moisture mozzarella cheese shredded
- 1 bell pepper, green, diced
- 1 oz. Can of sliced black olives, drained
- 16 pepperoni slices
- Oil

Directions

1. Build the dough (it can be completed ahead of time): Whisk together the flour, yeast, and salt

in a mixing bowl. Add water and oil. Mix the materials with a spoon or fork until dough develops. If it is too wet, add extra flour, then knead until a ball develops. Cover it and leave it to rest for 20 minutes. Use pre-made dough as an option.

2. Divide the dough into eight sections. Stretch and flatten the dough into nearly 4 ½ x 4 ½ inch squares while dealing for two pieces at a time.
3. Oil the pie iron and force it onto the bottom plate with one square of dough. Use the following ingredients: 2 tbsp of sauce, ¼ cup of cheese, ¼ of bell pepper, 1 oz of olives, and 4 pepperonis. Add a second square of dough to the top. Close & lock the iron for the pie.
4. Cook until the crust is golden brown, flipping if needed to assure even heat, over the flames or on top of your campfire embers. Depending on the campfire intensity, the precise time would be unpredictable, but usually, this will probably take 2-3 minutes. Check frequently.
5. Take from the heat, then open the pie iron properly and pull out the pizza pocket.
6. Repeat for the ingredients that left. Be conscious that when prepping additional pizza pockets, the iron will be HOT. Wait until the iron has cooled, or while reloading the iron, take extreme caution.

14. One-Pot Pesto Pasta with Bacon

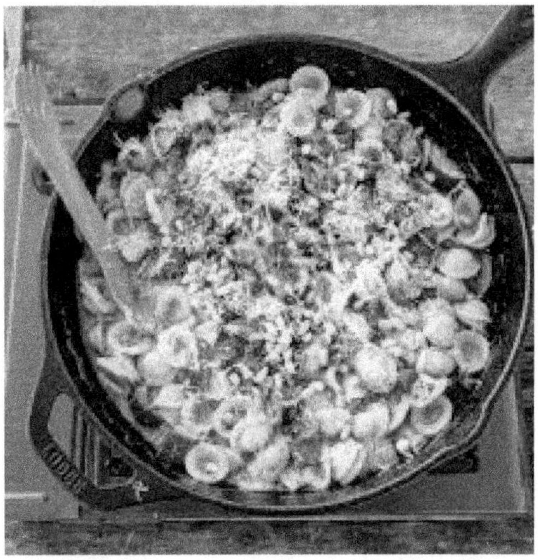

Serving: 2

Preparation time: 25 minutes

Nutritional values: 497kcal calories|52g carbohydrates|18g proteins|26g fat

Ingredients

- Bacon slices
- Zucchinis, diced
- A handful of cherry tomatoes
- 2 cups pasta
- 1/4 cup of pesto
- 1/4 cup of parmesan
- 2 tablespoons pine nuts
- Salt + pepper

Directions

1. In a skillet, cook the bacon over a moderate flame until crispy, then remove, cut, and set aside.
2. Add the zucchini, cherry tomatoes, and a bit of salt to the skillet and sauté for 5-7 minutes until the zucchini is soft and begins browning. Remove the vegetables and put them aside on a plate or bowl.
3. Transfer the pasta, 3 cups of water and half a teaspoon of salt to the skillet. Boil until the pasta is soft, and much of the water has been drained, stirring constantly-around 10 minutes (but check the packet directions). If needed, you may add more water, or if there is excess, dump at the top. Retract from the heat.
4. Integrate the pesto with the pasta, and add the vegetables, the parmesan cheese, the sliced bacon, and the pine nuts. Season with salt & pepper to taste. Enjoy.

15. Red Lentil Sloppy Joes

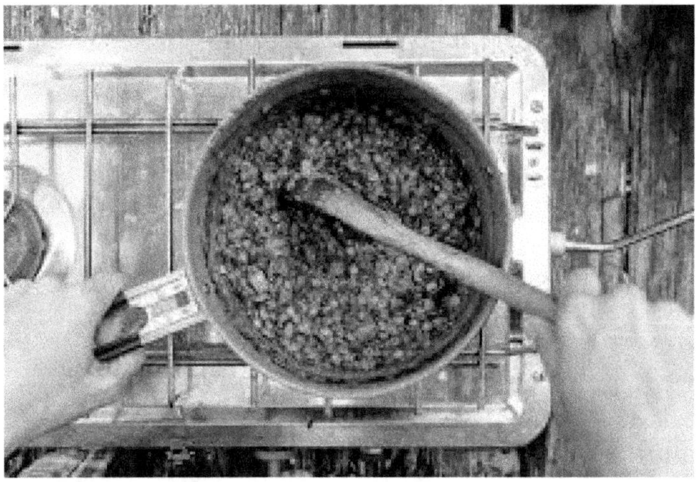

Serving: 2

Preparation time: 30 minutes

Nutritional values: 283kcal calories|7g carbohydrates|13g proteins|4g fat

Ingredients

- 1⁄2 teaspoons of oil
- 1 tiny onion, diced
- 1 pepper from Anaheim, diced tbsp tomato paste
- 2 teaspoons minced garlic
- 1⁄2 cup of red lentils
- 1 1⁄2 cup water or broth
- 1 tablespoon mustard
- 1 tablespoon of maple syrup
- 2 teaspoons of vinegar of apple cider
- 1 teaspoon Worcestershire vegan
- 1 teaspoon of chili powder
- 1⁄2 teaspoon of salt

Directions

1. Heat oil over medium temperature in a medium pot and add the sliced onions and Anaheim

pepper. Sauté for 3-4 minutes, until soft and the onions are just beginning to turn golden. Include the tomato paste, sauté for a minute, add the garlic and simmer for 1 minute.

2. To the pot, add the red lentils and 1 1/2 cup of water. Bring it to a boil, and let it simmer. Cook for 10-15 minutes, sporadically stirring, till the lentils are very soft but do not fall off.
3. Include mustard, maple syrup, apple cider vinegar, chili powder, Worcestershire, and salt. Stir to blend. Simmer until the sauce thickens a tad for 3-5 more minutes.
4. Serve with whatever toppings and sides you want, on toasted buns!

16. Campfire Grilled Fish Tacos with Spicy Corn Salsa

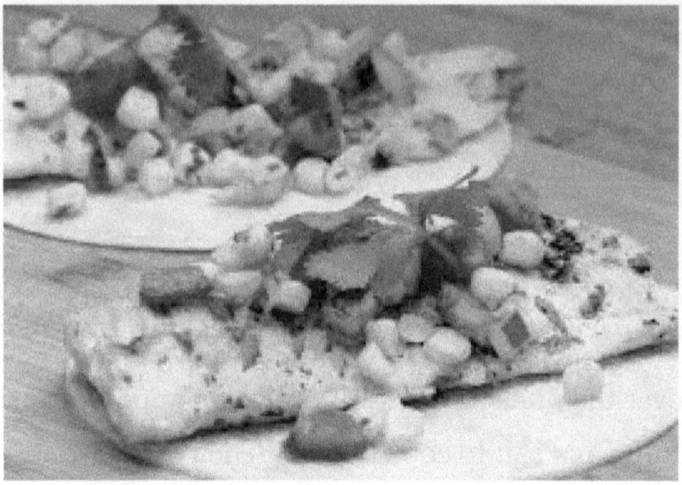

Serving: 6

Preparation time: 30 minutes

Nutritional values: 133kcal calories|9g carbohydrates|13g proteins|5g fat

Ingredients

For the Fish

- Snapper fillets or other white mild fish
- 1/2 lime
- 1 tablespoon of olive oil
- 1/2 tsp of salt
- 1 teaspoon of chili powder
- 1/2 teaspoon of cumin

For the Salsa Spicy Corn

- 1-2 ears of corn on a cob
- 1 jalapeno
- 1/2 tiny red onion
- 1/2 lime
- Handful of cilantro
- salt

To serve

- Six tortillas, warmed by the fire
- Hot sauce, optional
- Kettle Chips

Directions

1. Initiate your campfire or grill-this meal is going to be cooked over medium-high heat.
2. Squeeze half a lime over the fillets, drizzle with olive oil and then sprinkle all sides of the fish with chili powder, cumin, and salt to cook the fish. Then set aside.
3. Place the corn and jalapeno on the grill once your fire is set. Grill for about 10 minutes unless tender, rotating slightly. To cool somewhat, cut and put aside.
4. Place the fish in a basket with wire grills. Put and cook on the grill for around 3 minutes, then flip and cook for 2 more minutes. Remove and allow the fish to have a minute or two to relax.
5. Make the salsa when the fish is cooked. Cut the corn off the cob, peel off the jalapeno's blackened skin and chop (remove the stems & seeds for a milder spice), cut the onion thinly, and mince the cilantro. Put all in a bowl and squeeze half the lime into it. Add the salt as per your taste.
6. Use warmed tortillas, corn salsa, fish, and avocado to make your tacos. Serve and eat with a side of kettle chips.

17. Chicken and Potato Foil Packets

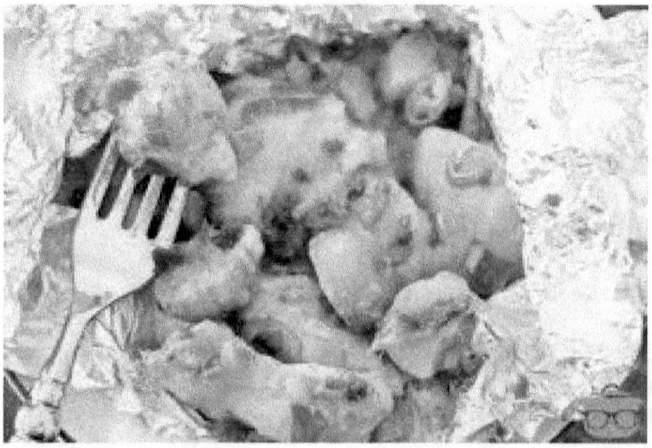

Serving: 4

Preparation time: 45 minutes

Nutritional values: 533kcal calories|59g carbohydrates|35g proteins|16g fat

Ingredients

- 1,1/2 pounds of finely cut baby potatoes
- 2 tbsp of olive oil
- 1 tbsp seasoning salt
- 1/4 tsp of pepper
- boneless chicken breasts, skinless
- 1/4 cup bacon pieces evenly
- 2/3 cup ground cheddar cheese
- 1 cup barbecue sauce, divided
- Green onions or chives
- 1 tbsp. sour cream, optional

Directions

1. Preheat the grill over medium heat.
2. Prepare packets of foil. Cover each with a broad piece of parchment paper (or coat with nonstick spray), then spread out 4 long pieces of heavy-duty foil.
3. In the center of each packet, placed equivalent numbers of sliced potatoes and onions. Add oil

and sprinkle with salt and pepper to taste.

4. Place the potatoes on top of the chicken breast. Using barbecue sauce to coat each side of the chicken breast.
5. By bringing 2 sides together and wrapping it out, wrap up every foil packet. Then, to secure the packet, roll up each open end.
6. Put on a hot grill and cook for around 25 minutes (potatoes down) or until juicy and chicken are grilled through (It should be 165 ° F).
7. Cover with cheddar cheese and bacon pieces, cut open packet, coat chicken with more BBQ sauce if required. Transfer to the grill (do not reseal) for around 5 minutes to melt.
8. Garnish with chives and sour cream

18. Camping Chicken Foil Dinner

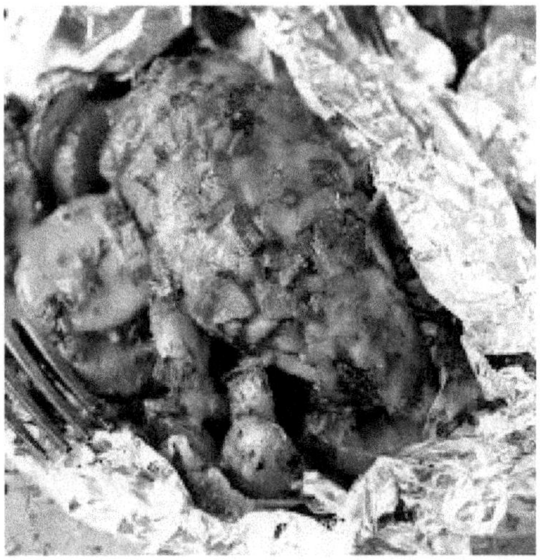

Serving: 4

Preparation time: 50 minutes

Nutritional values: 286kcal calories|42.8g carbohydrates|10.3g proteins|9.9g fat

Ingredients

- 4 large, heavy-duty or double-thick aluminum foil pieces
- Oil
- 4 tiny chopped potatoes
- 1 tiny chopped onion

- ears of corn (frozen cobs are okay) sliced in half
- Melted butter
- Basic spice rub or chosen spices
- boneless chicken thighs skinless, while using breasts, pound the thickest pieces flat.

Directions

To assemble:

1. Spread out the foil pieces and oil the centers of each of them.
2. Place the potatoes and onions in the middle of each piece of foil.
3. Brush the melted butter with the corn cobs and put them next to the potatoes. Slather your basic spice rub (or spices) with everything.
4. Atop the potatoes and onions, place the chicken and sprinkle with more seasoning rub.
5. Seal the edges tightly and nicely and leave a little space for steam. Place the packs in Ziplock baggies in case of leaking while taking to camping (which took place).
6. Cook or freeze for camping right away (use in the first 1-2 days).

In order to cook:

1. Cook frozen packets 5 inches from the fire/coals, on the one hand for 15 minutes and on the other for 15 minutes. While they are near to the campsites due to the stationary system, just switch them a little more often and shift them to prevent hot spots. In this situation, they may be cooked closer to the 20-minute mark, so after 15 minutes, you'll have to check.
2. It's all right if the packets are already partly frozen as you prepare them since they tend to cook over the hot campsite fire for the same period of time.
3. **Tip:** A few hours or days before, you can create packets for whatever fits your scheduling. You can also freeze them and cook partly thawed on the campsite afterward.

19. Sausage, Potato and Green Bean Foil Packets

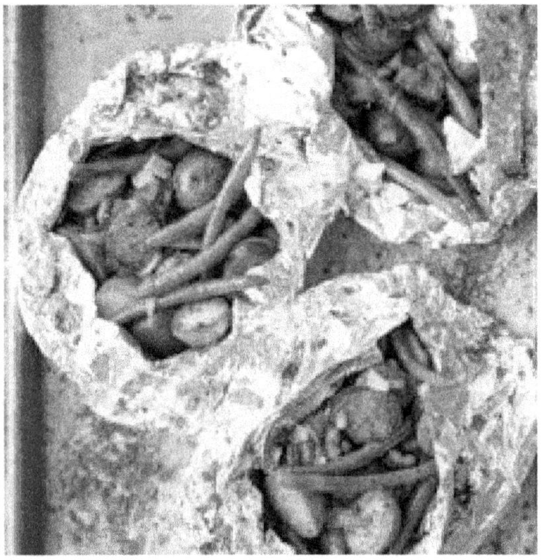

Serving: 4

Preparation time: 30 minutes

Nutritional values: 425.6kcal calories|34g carbohydrates|27.2g proteins|21g fat

Ingredients

- 1 (12.8-ounce) pack, smoked andouille sausage, thinly sliced
- 1 pound of baby red potatoes, sliced into quarters
- 1 pound of green, trimmed beans
- 2 Ounces of mushroom cremini halved
- 1 chopped onion
- 4 tbsp of unsalted, sliced butter
- 4 teaspoons of Cajun seasoning, cut
- Kosher salt and black pepper, freshly roasted, to taste
- 1 tbsp. of diced leaves of fresh parsley

Directions

1. Over extreme heat, preheat a gas or charcoal grill.
2. Cut four sheets of foil that are approximately 12 inches long. Divide the sausage, potatoes, green beans, mushrooms and onion into four equal portions and pertain a single layer to the

middle of the foil.

3. Fold up the 4 sides of each packet of foil. To your taste, add butter, Cajun seasoning, salt and pepper; gently toss to mix. Fold the sides of the foil over the sausage, cover and secure the closed packets entirely.
4. Put foil packets on the grill and cook for around 12-15 minutes until only cooked through.
5. Serve immediately, garnished with parsley, if required.

20. Campfire Cheesesteak

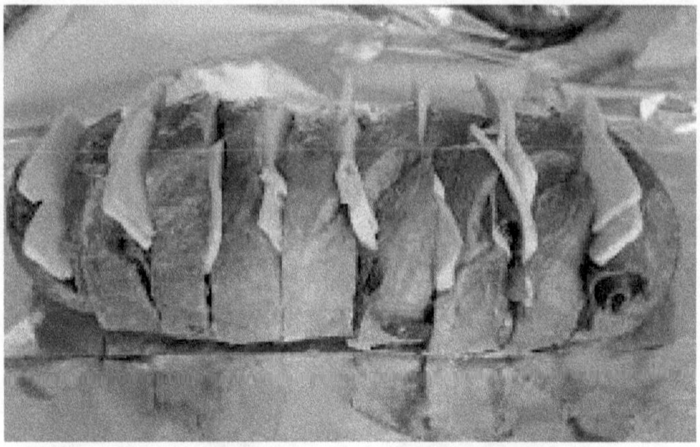

Serving: 4

Preparation time: 30 minutes

Nutritional values: 467kcal calories|23g carbohydrates|16g proteins|9g fat

Ingredients

- 1-pound roast beef sliced
- Onions
- Green peppers
- 1 loaf of bread with garlic
- Six pepper jack cheese slices
- 2 tablespoons of vegetable oil
- To taste, salt and pepper

Directions

1. Cut the onion and green peppers into strips. Before a camping trip, do this at home and store

it in a Ziplock container.

2. Heat oil over the fire in a pan.
3. While the oil is hot, add the onions and continue to cook until the browning begins.
4. Add the onions to the peppers and begin cooking until they are juicy and tender.
5. Place on the aluminum foil the open garlic bread and layer with roast beef.
6. While the onions and peppers have been cooked, put the roast beef on top.
7. On top of the onions and peppers, place all six slices of cheese.
8. On a sandwich, put the top slice of garlic bread and cover it with two layers of foil.
9. Place over or around the fire and cook for around 10 minutes or until the cheese melt.
10. Slice it into four pieces and eat it hot.

21. Grilled Potatoes

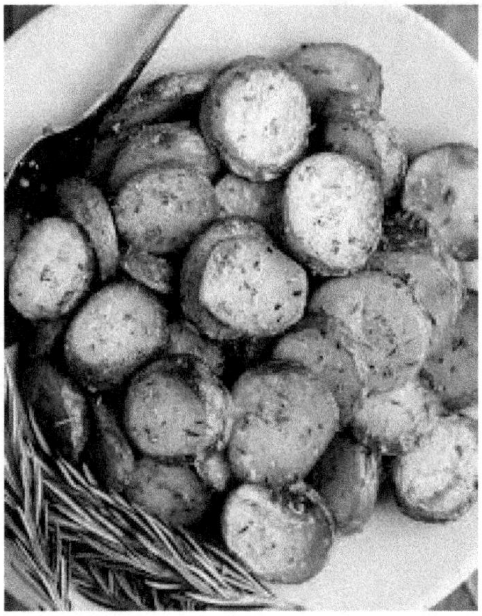

Serving: 4

Preparation time: 40 minutes

Nutritional values: 192kcal calories|37g carbohydrates|4g proteins|4g fat

Ingredients

- Red potatoes
- 1⁄4 cup olive oil

- Seasoning of potato
- 1 tsp rosemary
- 3/4 tsp oregano
- 3/4 teaspoons of thyme
- 3/4 teaspoons of sage
- 1/8 teaspoon of nutmeg
- 1 teaspoon salt
- 1/8 tsp of the pepper

Directions

1. For the potato seasoning, incorporate the spices. Drizzle much of the olive oil over the spice combination and mix well to combine. If needed, just add the leftover oil to the potatoes.
2. Slice the potatoes into slices that are 1/2 inch thick. Slice the circular ends thinly so that each side of the potato may stay flat on the grill.
3. In a large bowl, put the potato slices and drizzle them with the olive oil/seasoning blend. Toss it to coat properly.
4. Preheat to medium-high heat on the grill.
5. Two large sheets of foil are layered down and lightly sprayed with cooking spray.
6. Put the potatoes, if necessary, on top of the foil on a single sheet. Cover it with foil and close it.
7. On the grill, put the foil packet and close the lid. Heat for 20 minutes.
8. Using kitchen tongs to turn the potatoes and heat, uncovered, for an extra 5-10 minutes.
9. Remove from the grill and serve.

22. Camping Mac and Cheese with Kielbasa

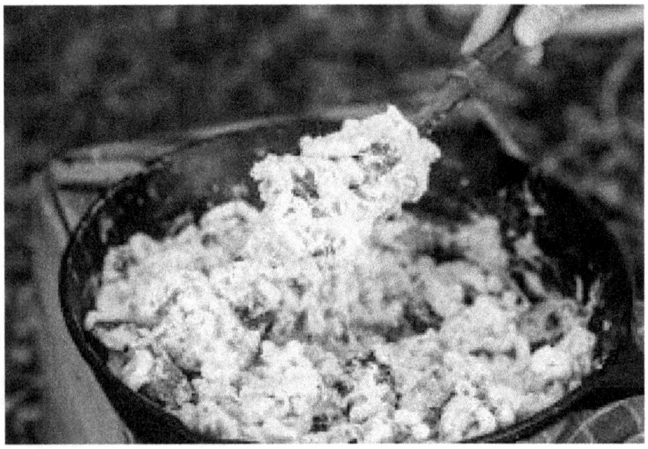

Serving: 8

Preparation time: 40 minutes

Nutritional values: 439kcal calories|14g carbohydrates|18g proteins|35g fat

Ingredients

- 1 kielbasa pack of 12-16 ounces, cut into 1-inch rounds
- 1 1/2 cups of noodles dry elbow macaroni
- 8-10 oz about 3/4 of a 15-ounce jar of Alfredo sauce
- 1 1/2 cup of cheddar and mozzarella shredded cheese combination, pizza blend or Mexican cheese blend
- 1/4-1/2 of a cup of milk
- For flavor, salt and pepper

Directions

1. Cook the kielbasa in a large cast-iron skillet or Dutch oven. Drain and set back any extra fat.
2. Cook the pasta according to product instructions in a separate pan. Dump with cold water and rinse. At home, you can cook noodles too, though. To end the cooking process, stun them with cold water and store them in a Ziplock bag in the cooler.
3. To make a sauce, add noodles, cheese, Alfredo sauce and add milk slowly (start with 1/4 of a cup and add more if necessary). Season with salt and pepper as per your taste.
4. Heat for 5-10 minutes on a grate over campfire coals, stirring periodically until the cheese is

fully melted.

5. Remove from the flames and instantly serve.

23. Camping Dutch Oven Chicken and Dumplings

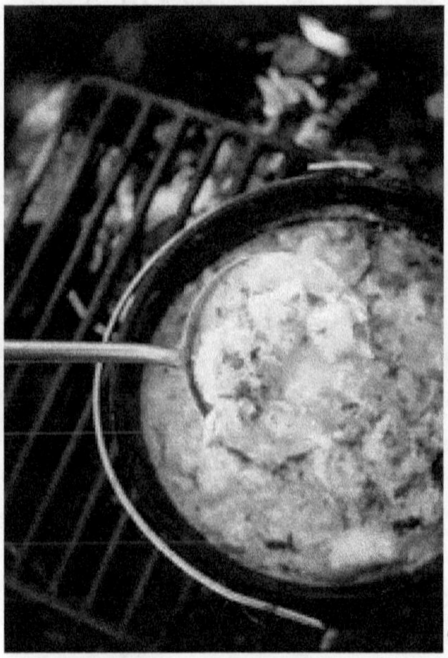

Serving: 8

Preparation time: 1 hour 20 minutes

Nutritional values: 49kcal calories|6g carbohydrates|3g proteins|2g fat

Ingredients

- 1 chicken broiler/fryer 2-1/2 to 3 pounds shredded or minced
- Three Cups of Water
- 1 cup onion chopped
- 4 celery ribs, diced
- medium carrots, diced
- 1 tsp seed celery
- 1 divided tsp. of rubbed sage
- 1 teaspoon of salt
- 1/4 of the pepper teaspoon
- cups of cookie/baking mix

- 3/4 of a cup plus two tbsp of milk
- 1 tablespoon fresh parsley minced

Directions

1. Put the water and chicken in a Dutch oven. Cover them and bring them to a boil.
2. Lower the heat to simmer; cook for around 30 minutes, until the chicken is tender.
3. Take the chicken out from the kettle, bone and cube.
4. Remove the carrot, celery, onions, celery seed, 1 tsp of sage, salt and pepper and transfer the chicken to the kettle.
5. Take it to a boil.
6. Minimize the heat.
7. For 45-60 minutes, cover and boil or until the vegetables are soft.
8. Integrate the biscuit mix, milk, parsley and residual sage to shape a stiff batter for dumplings or use a Can of biscuits.
9. Drop the tablespoonfuls into the chicken mixture that is simmering.
10. Close for 15 minutes and simmer.
11. Immediately serve and enjoy.

24. Cajun Shrimp Foil Packets

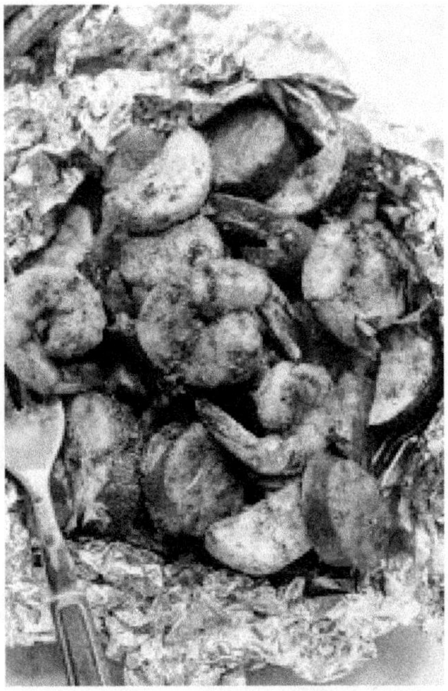

Serving: 4

Preparation time: 45 minutes

Nutritional values: 854kcal calories|62g carbohydrates|30g proteins|56g fat

Ingredients

- 18pieces of corn sticks (4 full corn sticks divided in half or quarter)
- 4 cleaned and diced red potatoes
- 25 uncooked peeled shrimp or not, the choice is yours
- 1 lb. of smoked sausage sliced into chunks
- 1/2 cup of melted olive oil or butter, as per your taste
- 1/2 cup of chicken potage, not needed much
- 1 Tbsp of Cajun/Creole topping, of Tony Chachere's brand to taste
- For flavor, salt and pepper

More elements to try (voluntary as to your taste) in a foil packet

- Sausages
- Chicken (cut the pieces into bite sizes)
- Bell Peppers
- Mushrooms
- Onions
- Celery
- Carrots

Directions

1. Heat a 400-degree grill. At the same temperature, you may even do this in the oven.
2. Spread the potatoes, corn, prawns, and sausages equally between 4 sheets of heavy foil (estimated 12x18 inches each).
3. Trickle the melted butter over each foil packet with around 2 tbsp of chicken potage.
4. With Cajun topping, pepper and salt, season uniformly and generously as per your taste.

5. Clamp the foil packs securely by folding the edges over the product and folding the ends tightly over the seam.
6. Grill for 35-40 minutes or until they become soft, tossing once halfway through the potatoes.
7. To check for readiness, be careful to open the packets; the steam present inside would be really hot.

3.3 Some Sweet Camping Recipes

1. Cherry Chocolate Pudgy Pie

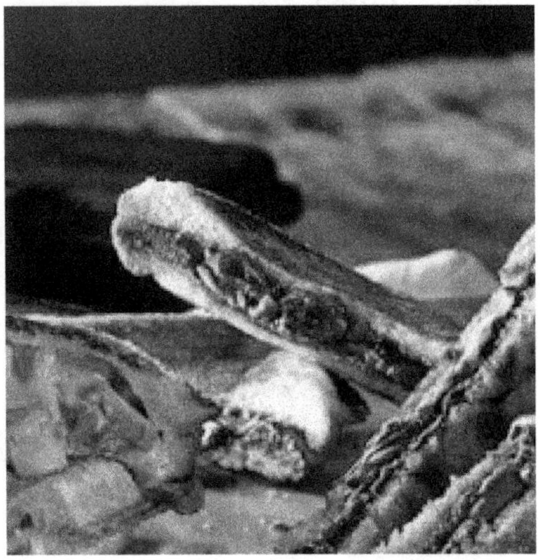

Serving: 1

Preparation time: 10 minutes

Nutritional values: 309kcal calories|51g carbohydrates|7g proteins|9g fat

Ingredients

- White bread slices
- 1 tbsp of cherry pie filling
- 1 tablespoon of almonds chopped
- 1 tablespoon of chocolate semisweet chips

Directions

1. Place 1 bread slice in the greased iron for the sandwich. Scattered with pie filling, top with chocolate chips, almonds and remaining slices of bread. Close the iron.

2. Cook until golden brown and cooked through, 3-6 minutes, rotating periodically over a hot campfire.

2. No-Bake Cereal Cookie Bars

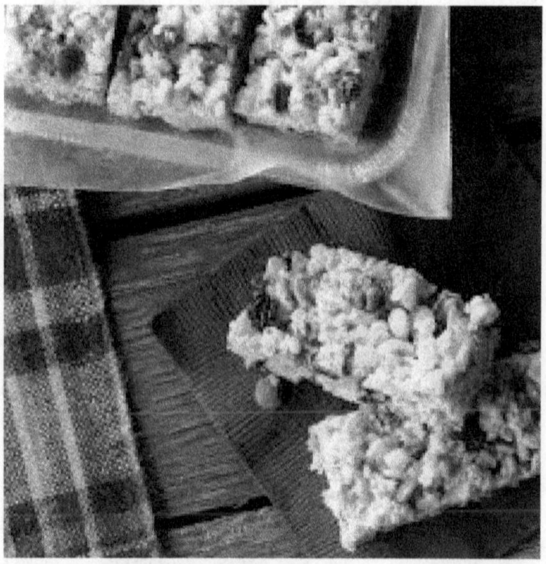

Serving: 3 dozen

Preparation time: 25 minutes

Nutritional values: 137kcal calories24g carbohydrates|2g proteins|4g fat

Ingredients

- 4-1/2 cups, Rice Krispies
- 3-1/4 cups of oats for quick-cooking
- 1/2 of a cup of cornflakes
- 1/2 cup shredded sweetened coconut
- 1/2 cup of butter, in cubes
- 1 package (16 ounces), Miniature Marshmallows
- 1/4 of a cup of honey
- 1/2 cup of M&M's minis
- 1/4 cup of berries

Directions

1. Grease a 15x10x1-in.pan. Combine the first 4 components in a wide bowl.
2. Melt butter over low heat in a large saucepan. Add the marshmallows; blend until completely melted. Incorporate honey unless mixed. Pour over the mixture of cereal; stir until uniformly covered. Cool for five minutes.
3. Whisk in M&M's and raisins; press a buttered spatula onto the prepared pan. Let it stand before cutting for 30 minutes. Place it in an airtight jar among layers of waxed paper.

3. Campfire Cinnamon Twists

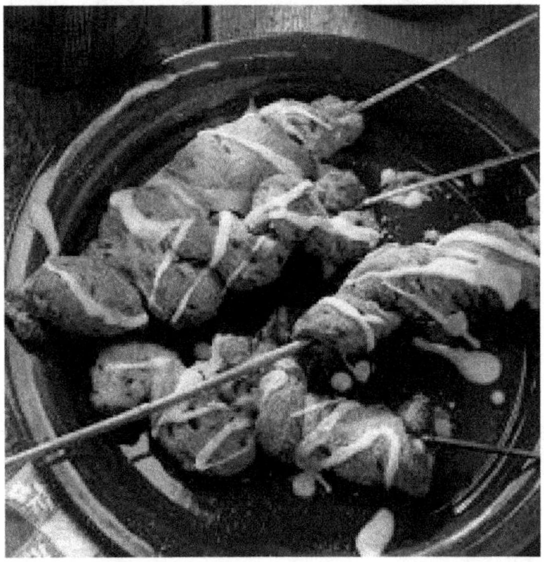

Serving: 16

Preparation time: 25 minutes

Nutritional values: 98kcal calories|15g carbohydrates|1g proteins|4g fat

Ingredients

- 1/4 cup of sugar
- 1 tsp. of ground cinnamon
- 1 tube of frozen cinnamon rolls with icing (12.4 ounces)
- 2 tablespoons of butter, melted

Directions

1. Integrate cinnamon and sugar. Remove the icing from the cinnamon rolls; transfer for dousing

to a resealable plastic bag.

2. Separate rolls; split in half, the each one. Roll into 6-in pieces, ropes. Wrap each rope firmly, beginning at 1/2 in, around a long metal skewer. Pointed end; pinch to protect each end.
3. Cook over a hot campfire for around 5 minutes, turning periodically, until golden brown. Sprinkle with butter; sprinkle with mixed sugar. Cut 1 corner of the icing bag through a narrow opening. Scatter the icing around the turns.

4. Campfire Pancakes with Peanut Maple Syrup

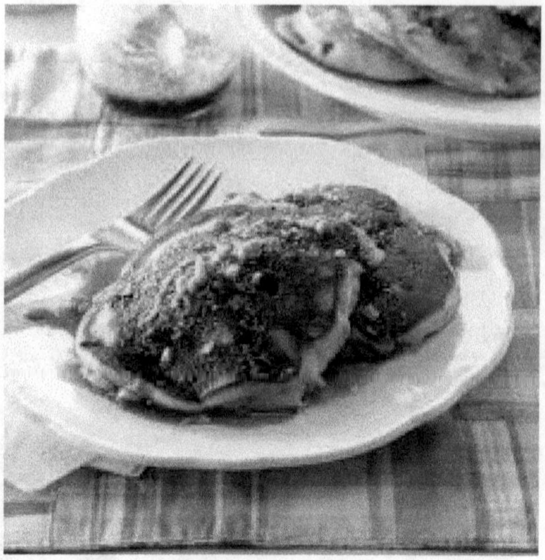

Serving: 8

Preparation time: 20 minutes

Nutritional values: 407kcal calories|63g carbohydrates|8g proteins|13g fat

Ingredients

- 1 box (6-1/2 ounces) muffin mix with chocolate chips
- 2/3 cup of 2% milk
- 1 large egg, beaten lightly
- 1/2 cup miniature marshmallows
- 1/4 cup chips of butterscotch
- 1/4 cup syrup of maple
- 1 tbsp chunky peanut butter

Directions

1. Combine the muffin mix, milk and egg in a wide bowl; whisk until moistened. Fold in the chips and marshmallows.
2. Grease a griddle lightly; place it over moderate flame. Pour 1/4 of a cupful of batter onto the griddle. Cook until the top bubbles are appearing, and the bottoms are nicely browned. Turn over; cook until golden brown on the second side.
3. Meanwhile, when cooked through, heat maple syrup and peanut butter at 10- to 20-second intervals. Serve with pancakes.

5. Éclairs on the Grill

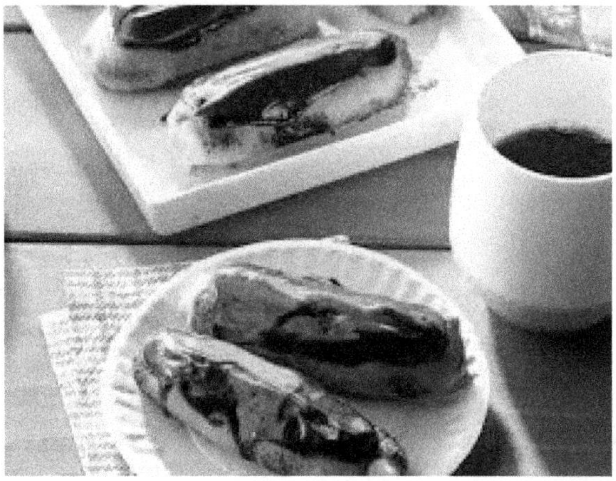

Serving: 6

Preparation time: 10 minutes

Nutritional values: 293kcal calories|43g carbohydrates|4g proteins|12g fat

Ingredients

- Wooden dowel or stick (5/8-inch diameter and 24-inch long)
- 1 tube (8 ounces) seamless refrigerated crescent dough layer
- snack-size cups of vanilla or chocolate pudding (3-1/4 ounces each)
- 1/2 cup frosting of chocolate
- Can of whipped cream

Directions

1. Get your campfire or grill set for high heat. Use foil to cover one side of a stick or wooden dowel.

Unroll the crescent dough and split it into six 4-in squares. Wrap the prepared stick around one slice of dough; pinch the end and seam to secure.

2. Cook for 5-7 minutes over a campfire or grill or until lightly browned, turning frequently. Remove from the stick until the dough is cold enough to handle. Cooling is done. Repeat for the dough that is left.
3. Place the pudding in a Ziploc bag; at one corner, cut a tiny opening. Squeeze the bag onto each shell and press the mixture into it. Use frosting to spread and top with whipped cream.

Conclusion

Camping is an ideal way to enjoy fantastic local produce. The best food and drink for camping involves various things to different individuals (and differs widely based on whether you are camping in a vehicle or backpacking). Picnics and camping are generally a bit better, since if it's already done, you're only transporting it, but preparing a great meal while camping is not that challenging, as long as you meet certain general instructions. Probably your home kitchen has a freezer, pantry, sufficient cabinets and quick access to a nearby supermarket where thousands of choices are accessible for any meal. However, the camping kitchen of yours is a little more mounted down, perhaps limited to a cooler, storage box, plastic jar/container or two, and perhaps a weekend bag made of paper that remains in your car's backseat.

The natural wood smoke gives any dish an amazing taste, whilst the gentle crackle of flames enables campfire cooking a relaxing way to experience the great outdoors. However, you don't have to associate fewer ingredients on hand with dull recipes, especially when you realize how some main staples will blend in dozens of ways, if not hundreds, enabling you to cook up dishes to please a lonely hiker, a romantic couple, a starving family, as well as a whole crowd sitting across the campfire.

It is probably better to make all food planning you can do as minimal as possible while camping. Minimize the use of perishable food products and follow the proper sanitation precautions to ensure your group members' welfare. However, that picnic and cookouts are a feature of the camping culture. For this purpose, it is important to take care of all the precautions. There are a few food planning staples that you shouldn't skip, regardless of whether you intend to prepare for your upcoming camping trip or hiking. A case of matches and some fluid used as a firelighter are first and foremost.

The majority tend to cook over an outdoor fire at their campsite, so you'd be not so lucky without the need for a means to start one. For the dishes, a medium-sized to large-sized lightweight bowl, a similar size skillet, foil of aluminum, and a compact grill that can be put over a fire grate are the real necessities. This variation of cooking appliances helps produce Ham, eggs, lentils, and pasta. Finally, don't skip your spatula and tongs. It's far from enjoyable to pull food from a bare-handed fire.

Book 2:Dash Diet Cookbook

Quick and Easy Recipes to Rapidly Reduce Hypertension

Introduction

Hypertension remains the most important cause of death worldwide. But via therapy and dietary change, it is preventable. Hypertension management methods consist of dietary modifications including a diet high in fruits, low-fat foods or fish and vegetables with a reduced saturated and total fat content, limited salt intake, regular exercise, appropriate body weight, less alcohol consumption, and drug therapies, even though these differ to some extent according to various published treatment guidelines for hypertension.

Starting the DASH diet is one of the moves your doctor might prescribe to reduce your high blood pressure.

DASH is abbreviated as "Dietary approaches to stop hypertension". The DASH diet is intended to treat or avoid elevated blood pressure (hypertension) and is a comprehensive strategy to have healthy nutrition. In studies funded by the National Institutes of Health, the DASH diet strategy was designed to reduce blood pressure without medicine. Vegetables and low-fat dairy foods are favored in the DASH diet, as well as the optimum number of whole grains, poultry, nuts and fishes.

There is also a reduced salt variant of the diet, in addition to the regular DASH diet. You should pick the diet variant that suits your requirements for health.

The DASH diet helps you lower the sodium concentration in the daily routine diet and enables you to enjoy several nutrient-rich foods that contain potassium, magnesium and calcium to lower the blood pressure.

You could be able to reduce the blood pressure by a few steps in approximately two weeks by adopting the DASH diet. Your high blood pressure (the systolic) can decrease by 8 - 14 points with the time that can make a considerable difference to your health risks.

Since the DASH diet is a safe way of eating, it not only reduces blood pressure but also provides cardiovascular benefits.

For the treatment of cancer, osteoporosis, heart disease, diabetes and stroke, the DASH diet is also in suggestion with nutritional guidelines.

Chapter 1 – DASH Diet

1.1 Origin

Dietary Methods to avoid Hypertension (DASH) emerged in the 1990s. The National Institute of Health (NIH) began funding a variety of research studies in 1992 to see that particular dietary approaches are effective in the treatment of hypertension or not. To prevent any potential factors, the study participants were recommended to follow only the dietary treatments and not include any other lifestyle changes. They observed that systolic blood pressure could only be lowered by around 6 to 11 mmHg by dietary activity alone. This influence was shown in persons with both hypertension and normotension. In several cases, the DASH diet centered upon these findings has been advised as the first-line therapy with a lifestyle change.

1.2 What is used in this diet?

DASH encourages the intake of fruits, vegetables, lean meat and milk items and the use of micronutrients in the menu. The lowering of sodium in the diet to around 1500 mg/day is often advocated. DASH focuses on the consumption of food that is minimally refined and fresh. There are also similarities between the DASH diet and some of the other nutritional strategies advocated for cardiovascular fitness. The DASH diet is an apogee of the modern world, as well as ancient times. Scientists have mined it on the basis of some ancient culinary principles, and it has been adapted to target some of the leading causes of mortality and morbidity in the modern world.

1.3 Enhancing Healthcare Team Outcomes

For controlling hypertension, the DASH diet is a nutritionally balanced approach. In many clinical trials, the diet has been studied and found to reduce saturated fats, blood pressure and cholesterol. DASH diet has been prescribed as the safest diet for those who wish to lose weight and reduce blood pressure. The real criterion is that the patients must be encouraged to this diet. Both nurses and pharmacists play a vital role in teaching the patients about the effects of this diet in addition to doctors. Nurses are in a perfect role. They can teach both patients and family members more about the DASH diet and its advantages right before discharge.

Similarly, the pharmacist should teach the customer about the DASH diet while patients visit a

pharmacy. The DASH diet's most critical features are that it needs a lifestyle transition and a healthier way to eat. In conjunction, patients should be advised to avoid smoking, refrain from alcohol, and actively engage in any physical exercise.

1.4 Is the DASH diet primarily preferred for Hypertension care only?

It has been researched thoroughly to check the DASH diet's treatment paradigm and its effects on several other diseases.

Several studies have found that the DASH diet improves by reducing triglycerides, LDL-C, blood glucose levels, as well as insulin tolerance. Such behavior allows the DASH diet to significantly contribute to metabolic syndrome's pharmacological treatment (a major epidemic in this region). It has also become a powerful element for weight control. Complying some populations with the DASH diet has demonstrated substantial changes in type 2 diabetes treatment. Its focus on lowering dietary sodium and promoting the consumption of calcium, potassium, and magnesium, which is a recommended diet in patients with heart disease.

1.5 Research and general acceptance

Reports have indicated that excessive salt consumption plays a role in high blood pressure progression over the years. Dietary recommendations for the avoidance and control of hypertension have mostly centered on reducing sodium or salt consumption. In 1989, a study scrutinized the reaction of 3 to12 g of salt consumption per day to blood pressure. This study showed that a small decrease in salt, i.e., 5-6 g of salt a day, allows the blood pressure to decrease in patients with hypertension. The better result was shown with just 3 g of salt a day intake, with a mean drop in blood pressure of systolic (11 mmHg) and diastolic (6 mmHg), respectively. More notably, the low-salt diets used for high blood pressure reduction or recovery have been questioned. The Phase II Hypertension Prevention Trials in 1997 suggested that energy consumption and weight loss in the prevention of hypertension were more significant than limiting dietary salt. A 2006 Cochrane study (which investigated the effect of a longer-term moderate reduction in salt on blood pressure) observed that a modest decrease in salt consumption could substantially influence blood pressure in individuals with hypertension but a smaller impact on those without blood pressure. It was decided that the 2007 public health

guidelines would have a positive impact on blood pressure and cardiovascular disease by reducing salt consumption from 9-12 g / day to a modest level i.e., 5-6 g /day.

The potency of a DASH diet is well known for controlling blood pressure. As an example of a healthy eating schedule (compatible with the 2015 Dietary Guidelines' current recommendations for Americans), proposed the DASH Eating Plan, which constitutes the foundation for USDA MyPlate and their recommendations, such as those promoted by a British Nutrition Foundation, American Society for Hypertension and the American Heart Association also prescribe the DASH.

While lowering sodium and increasing the consumption of potassium, calcium, and magnesium play a crucial role in decreasing blood pressure, but the reasons for the beneficial effects of the DASH eating plan remain unclear. The researchers say that it may be that whole food ingests potassium, calcium, and magnesium, or it may be due to the combined effect of consuming those nutrients collectively rather than the specific nutrients individually. It is also suspected that the link between diet and blood pressure could be another anonymous factor present in fruits, vegetables, and low-fat dairy products.

The Salt Institute encourages the DASH diet but without limiting the salt. They assert that a DASH diet alone would produce the necessary decrease in blood pressure without the decreased sodium consumption from packaged foods. Their suggestion is focused on the reality that no evidence-based findings justify a need for the whole population to limit dietary salt. The 2006 Cochrane review found that a small decrease in salt consumption dramatically reduce blood pressure in hypertension's patient but had little impact on average blood pressure. The salt limitation is not advised for people without hypertension.

1.6 Precautions

To prevent side effects such as gas, bloating, and diarrhea, the addition of high-fiber foods to the diet should be achieved progressively. Increasing fluid at the same time is necessary since fiber pulls water into the intestine. High fibers consumption can induce hard stools and constipation with insufficient fluid.

The rise in fruits and vegetables improves the diet's potassium content. A higher intake of potassium from foods presents little risk for healthy people with proper kidney function because

extra potassium is excreted in the urine. However, there may be a chance of hyperkalemia (high potassium levels in the blood) in people whose urinary potassium excretion is compromised, such as patients with end-stage renal disease, significant cardiac failure or adrenal insufficiency. Hyperkalemia can lead to an erratic heartbeat (cardiac arrhythmia), which can be dangerous. Also, some popular medications may minimize the excretion of potassium. Before beginning the DASH diet, patients at risk should contact a doctor since a higher intake of potassium in the form of fruit and vegetables might not be sufficient. For the substitution of potassium-containing salt, caution should also be taken.

1.7 Risks

There are no known complications linked with the DASH diet currently. The long-term impacts of the diet on illness and mortality are still uncertain.

Chapter 2 – Sample menus for the DASH diet

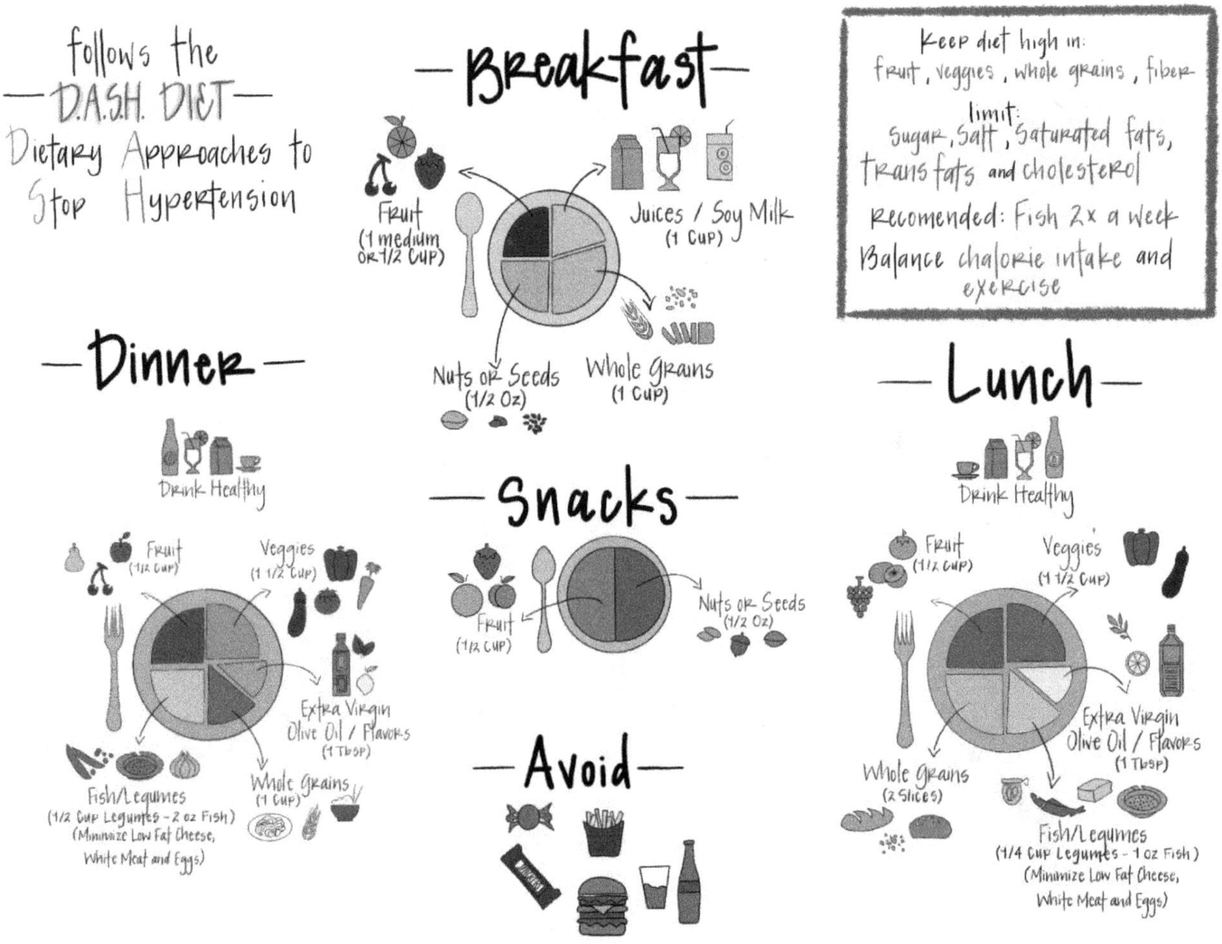

2.1 Involved in implementing the eating schedule for DASH, but how?

The DASH diet includes menus containing whole foods, seafood, meat and nuts, lots of greens, fruits and low-fat dairy products. Small portions of red meat, desserts and drinks are also offered.

You may like to try the DASH diet, but you're not sure how to combine DASH into your regular menus. Here are the menus, conforming to the DASH schedule to help you get started. As a basis for your balanced meal plans, use these menus.

Remember that you may eat a few more or a few smaller portions on certain days than prescribed for a specific food category. That's normally fine, as far as the guidelines are similar to the average of a few days or even a week. The exception is that of sodium. Aim to remain as close to the daily sodium level as possible. Notice also that nutritional content values can differ based on the particular brands of ingredients you use or alterations you make in preparing meals.

Formulating the DASH diet aims to reduce blood pressure and to diminish the risk of heart disease. In developed nations, heart disease remains the leading cause of death in males and females, and meaningful actions can be taken to significantly decrease its chances.

That's because all of the heart disease risk factors are largely within our control. They include actively participating in inappropriate exercise, preventing obesity and eating a balanced diet. For starters, merely removing added sugars from the diet will reduce the risk. It can also greatly impact your risk profile by eating more fruits, vegetables and whole grains and eating less refined and red meat. Too many sugars and too much meat intake is associated with reduced health. Conversely, it would be helpful to replace these ingredients with more nutritious substitutes.

Persons using the DASH diet in clinical trials decreased their blood pressure after two weeks. Another diet, DASH-Sodium, allows sodium to be downsized to 1,500 mg per day (approximately 2/3 of a teaspoon). Studies of individuals on the DASH-Sodium diet have reduced their blood pressure.

Starting the DASH Diet: The DASH diet needs a few numbers of daily servings from different food groups. Depending on the number of calories you require each day, the number of servings can vary that you need. It would be best if you made incremental alterations. For example: start by restricting yourself to 2400 mg of sodium a day (about one teaspoon). Then, cut down to 1500 mg of sodium a day (about 2/3 teaspoons) until the body transitions to the diet. These levels include all absorbed sodium, including sodium consumed in food items and fried things or added to the table.

2.2 Dash Diet Tips

- Add servings of vegetables in lunch and dinner.
- For your dinners or as a snack, add servings of fruit.
- It is quick to use canned and dried fruits, but ensure that they have no added sugar.
- Using just half the traditional butter, salad dressing, margarine serving, and low or fat-free seasonings.
- Drink low-fat or skim dairy items whenever you use cream or full-fat.
- Limit meat to 6 ounces a day. Make some vegetable meals.
- Drink low-fat or skim dairy items where full-fat or cream is usually used.

- Restrict the amount of meat to 6 ounces daily.
- Have some veggie meals.
- Add more dried beans and fruits to your daily diet.
- Eat unsalted pretzels or almonds, raisins, reduced sugar and fat-free milk, unsalted, plain popcorn without butter, fresh veggies and frozen yogurt instead of snacking sweets and chips.
- To select items that are lower in sodium, read the food labels.

2.4 To continue the DASH Diet

The DASH diet recommends to get:

Grains: 7 to 8 daily servings

Vegetables: 4 to 5 daily servings

Fruits: 4 to 5 daily servings

Low or fat-free milk products: 2 to 3 daily servings

Meat, fish and poultry: 2 or <2 servings

Seeds, nuts and dry beans: 4 to 5 servings a week

Oils and Fats: 2 to 3 daily servings

Sweets: tend to limit < 5 servings a week

Below is a closer look at those guidelines.

Carbohydrates:

Carbohydrates are mostly made up of cellulose and starches in the diet. The human body cannot digest cellulose. It is predominantly found in fiber from plants. In the diet, "carbs" or healthy starches must be included, not just for the availability of calories but also for the defensive micronutrients. Low carb diets are not as safe as this will result in lowered calorie consumption as prescribed or an additional intake of unhealthy fats.

Under DASH, balanced carbohydrates include:

- **Green leafy vegetables: kale, broccoli, spinach, collards and mustards**
- **Legumes and beans**

- **Low glucose index fruits**
- **Whole grains: millets, cracked wheat and oats**

Fats:

Fats are a prime suspect in the advancement of the chronic disease epidemic most of the time. However, research has now proven true. Fats are now classified as good and bad fats.

Good fats supply essential fatty acids, promote overall health and avoid inflammation. These fats have increased HDL and decreased small, dense LDL particles when consumed in moderation. Some of the sources of good fats also included in DASH include:

- **Avocados**
- **Fish rich in omega-3 fatty acids**
- **Flax seeds**
- **Hempseeds**
- **Nuts**
- **Olive oil**

Bad fats, including vegetable shortenings, margarine, partly hydrogenated vegetable oils, induce an increase in atherogenesis-promoting minor LDL particles.

Fats are a heavily concentrated energy supply that has to be eaten in moderation. Thus their serving amounts in the DASH guidelines are much lower than those for other nutrients.

Proteins:

More servings of plant proteins, including soy products, legumes, seeds and nuts, are advised by DASH. In the diet, animal protein can primarily consist of lean meats, eggs, low-fat milk products, and fish. Since they have been shown to induce hypertension and even contain carcinogens, therefore, cured and dried meats are not suggested.

The DASH diet also addresses the use of some foods high in potassium, magnesium and calcium, as they inhibit endothelial dysfunction and facilitate endothelial relaxing of the smooth muscle. Bananas, Spinach and oranges are some of the potassium-rich foods. Calcium is rich in green leafy vegetables and dairy products. In several leafy greens, whole grains, beans and nuts, magnesium is present.

2.3 Change gradually

Add a serving at lunch and another at dinner if you are eating one or two vegetables a day. Add a serving to your meals or have it as a snack, if you do not eat fruit or have only juice at breakfast. Improve your use of fat-free and low-fat milk and milk products gradually to 3 servings a day. Drink milk at lunch or at dinner instead of sugar-sweetened tea, soda or alcohol. To reduce your consumption of saturated fat, the total fat, cholesterol, and calories and boost your calcium, choose fat-free (skimmed) or low fat (1 %) milk products. To choose the lowest saturated fat and trans-fat, read the nutrition facts on salad dressings and margarine.

2.5 Making the DASH to Good Health

A new way of eating for a lifetime is the DASH plan. Don't let it away from accessing your fitness goals if you slip out of the diet pattern for a few days. Return to the track.

Here's how:

Ask yourself why you have been off-track. Has it been at a party? Were you at home or work and feeling stressed? Find out how you divagated and start with the DASH plan again. Yes, don't worry about slipping. Especially when learning something new, everybody slips. Remember that it is a long-term process to change your lifestyle. See if you've tried to do too much all at once. Those who are beginning a new lifestyle often try to change too much at once. Change one or two things at a time instead. It is the best way to succeed, slowly but surely. Break down the cycle into small steps. By doing so, you will not only be stopped to execute excessively at once, but it also makes the modifications simpler. Break complicated objectives into smaller and simpler steps, and each of which is achievable. Write down that. To keep a record of your eaten food and what you're doing. This activity can assist you in finding the issue. Keep track of multiple days. For example, you may find that while watching television, you eat high-fat foods. If so, instead of high-fat foods, you could start keeping a substituted snack on hand to eat. This record also helps you be sure that you get enough of every food group and physical activity every day. Celebrate performance. For your achievements, treat yourselves to a non-food treat.

Chapter 3 – Breakfast Recipes

New literature indicates that eating a too much breakfast, a more moderate lunch, and consuming less meal at dinner time is an eating plan associated with improved weight loss and management for individuals trying to lose (or control) body weight. When we eat most of our daily calories early in the day, it appears we fare better.

In the face of the experiences and traditions of other Americans, this travels. On the run, we prefer to eat breakfast and leave the big meal for the day's end. A safer approach is there. Why not try and eat the most of your calories and allow yourself to enjoy your feast in the morning?

To help you live a healthy life, the DASH Diet focuses on ingredients consumption in the morning to reduce your blood pressure. A significant tip is here: Never, ever, miss breakfast. It is counter-productive, and later in the day, it sets you up for overeating. By choosing a nutritional breakfast to eat, launch your day right off. In this diet plan, healthy breakfast selections include protein, fruits, vegetables, low-fat dairy products and whole grains. Give a lift to your mornings with these delectable recipes.

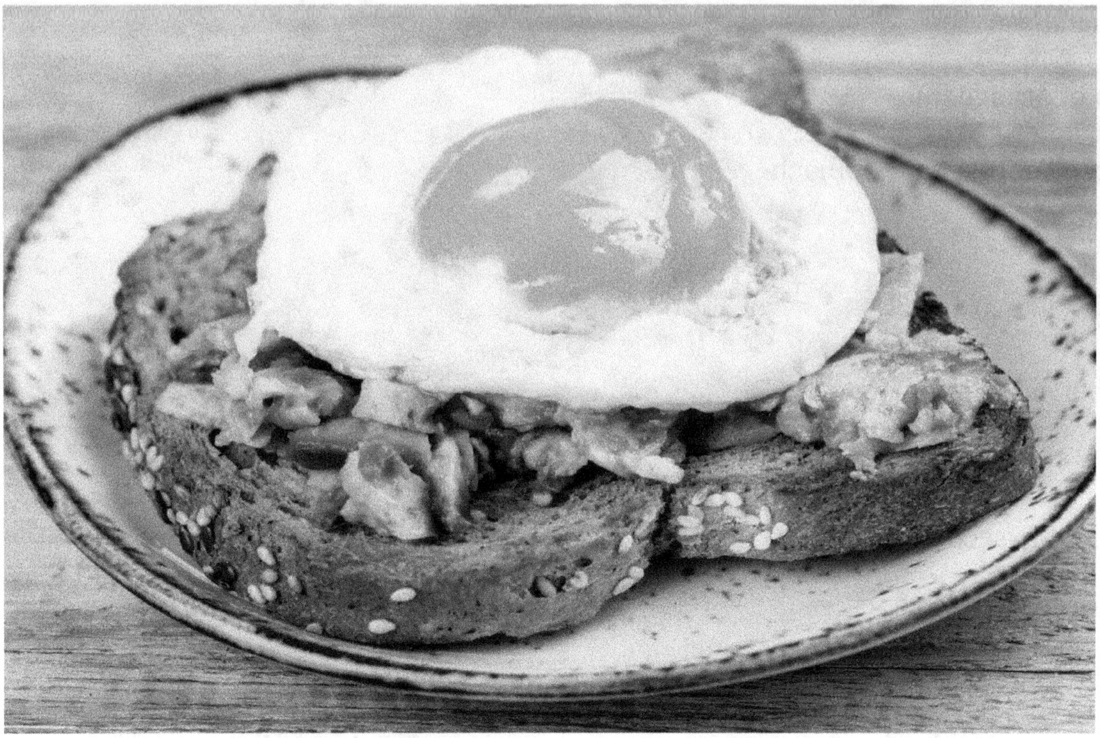

3.1 Almond Butter Berry Smoothie

YIELD: 2 servings

Ingredients

- 1 tablespoon almond butter (creamy)
- 1 cup fresh/frozen raspberries
- 1/2 medium banana (ripe)
- 1/2 cup ice (crushed)
- 1/4 cup low-fat milk (1%)

Directions

Blend until smooth, and then enjoy all the ingredients.

3.2 Spinach Sunshine Smoothie Bowl

YIELD: 1 serving

Ingredients

- 1 banana
- 1 cup of orange juice
- 1 packed cup of baby spinach
- 1/2 avocado
- 1/2 cup of ice cubes
- blueberries (optional)
- diced pineapple (optional)
- ground flaxseeds (optional)

Directions

1. Cook the spinach, avocado, pineapple, orange juice, and ice until it becomes creamy.
2. Filled with sliced ground flaxseeds, pineapple and blueberries and serve.

3.3 Peaches And Pomegranate Avocado Toast

YIELD: 1 serving

Ingredients

- 1 slice of whole-grain bread
- 1 teaspoon ricotta
- pomegranate seeds(small handful)
- honey drizzles
- 1/2 avocado

Directions

1. In the microwave oven or toaster, toast the whole grain bread.
2. Spread avocado (coarse or smooth as you want) on the toast.
3. Spread all over the avocado with a dollop of ricotta.
4. Drizzle over the avocado mixture with a touch of butter.
5. Sprinkle on top of pomegranate seeds and enjoy.

3.4 Breakfast in a Jar

YIELD: 1 serving

Ingredients

- 1 tablespoon of chia seeds
- 2 tablespoon raisins
- 1 tablespoon unsweetened coconut flakes
- 1/4 cup of oatmeal
- 3/4 cup of kefir

Directions:

1. In a 16-ounce mason jar, cover the ingredients, cover the lid, and keep in refrigerate overnight.
2. Take the container from the fridge when it's time to eat and give it a fast stir.

3.5 Avocado Egg Cups

YIELD: 4 servings

Ingredients

- 2 avocados (ripened)
- 4 medium eggs
- 1 tablespoon of grated cheese (like Parmesan, Swiss or cheddar)
- 1/2 tablespoon of olive oil
- 1/4 tablespoon of coarse salt
- 1/4 tablespoon of pepper

Assorted toppings: scallions, herbs, salsa, diced tomato, Sriracha, paprika, crumbled bacon and crumbled feta

Directions:

1. Heat the oven to 375 °F. Halve the avocados and pit lengthwise. Cut a quite thin slice from the bottom of each half of the avocado such that the level lies. Scoop out enough of the flesh (around ½ tbsp) and pit it, inorder to make space for an egg.

2. Place the avocados on a rimmed baking sheet lined with foil. Season with pepper and salt, and apply the olive oil to the mixture.

3. Through each cavity, smash an egg (some of the white egg will run over the side, so don't think about it). Sprinkle (if used) with cheese. Cover with foil loosely.

4. Bake for 20 to 25 minutes or until you have your eggs prepared to your taste. And sprinkle with toppings.

3.6 Daphne Oz's Sugar Break Apple and Peanut Butter Oatmeal

YIELD: 4 servings

Ingredients

- 1 cup of steel-cut oats
- peanut butter's swirl

- pinch ground cinnamon
- 1 tablespoon butter (optional)
- 4 cups of water
- Pinch of salt
- 3 medium of large Granny Smith apples (cored and sliced into 1 or 2-inch chunks)

Directions:

1. Process the oats until they hit the thickness and creaminess at the desired level.

2. Chop the apples and toss them with the oats, and then stir.

3. Attach the peanut butter and stir until it is melted and spread all over.

4. Cover the cinnamon and butter with a splash (not mandatory) and enjoy it.

3.7 Sweet Potato Toast

YIELD: 1 serving

Ingredients

- 1 potato (sweet)

Directions

1. Cut into 1/4-inch slices of the sweet potato and put it in the toaster.

2. Top that with anything you want. Nut butter with strawberries, avocado, hummus, eggs, cheese, and tuna salad are common combos.

Note: The amount of calories is based on one sweet potato but does not consider the toppings.

Various toppings will add 25-383 extra calories everywhere. Cut the sweet potato into 1/4-inch slices and pop into the toaster.

3.8 Tofu Turmeric Scramble

YIELD: 2 servings

Ingredients

- ¼ cup of nutritional yeast

- ¼ red onion (chopped)
- ½ cup button mushrooms (sliced)
- ½ tablespoon turmeric
- ½ tablespoon of salt and pepper
- 1 8-ounce block of firm/extra-firm tofu (drained)
- 1 green or red bell pepper (chopped)
- olive oil (extra virgin)
- garlic powder
- 2 cups fresh Spinach (loosely chopped)

Directions

1. To eliminate excess water, clear the tofu and pinch gently. Crumble the tofu by hand into a bowl-the finer pieces will be better.

2. Put a large skillet on medium heat and cook the vegetables. Include the olive oil, onions, and bell peppers when ready. Mix a pinch of the pepper and salt and simmer to soften the vegetables for around 5 minutes. Add the mushrooms and stir-fry for 2 minutes. Add tofu then. Stir-fry for 3 minutes or slightly longer if the tofu is thin.

3. Then add the remaining salt & pepper, garlic, nutritional yeast and turmeric and mix well with a spatula to ensure that spices are well balanced. Cook until the tofu is finely browned, for another 5 to 8 minutes.

4. Add the Spinach and steam for 2 minutes to coat the pan. Serve instantly.

3.9 Ulli's Granelli

YIELD: 26 servings

Ingredients

- 1/2 cup of maple syrup
- 1/3 cup orange oil (pure)
- 1/4 cup coconut oil (unrefined), along with 2 tablespoon for oiling the baking sheet

- 2 cups dried cherries/cranberries
- 2 cups raisins (organic)
- 2 cups almonds (raw)
- 2 cups cashews (raw)
- 2 cups pumpkin seeds (raw)
- 2 cups sunflower seeds (raw)
- 2 cups walnuts (raw)
- 3 cups unsweetened coconut flakes
- 4 cups rolled oats
- pinch of sea salt

Directions

1. Preheat the Microwave oven to 300 degrees Fahrenheit.

2. Combine the peas, almonds, seeds and coconut flakes in a large bowl and blend well.

3. Whisk the maple syrup, salt and coconut oil and orange oil together in a smaller bowl until thoroughly mixed, then spill over the oat-nut mixture and meld well.

4. Spread granola on a large oiled baking sheet (do it in batches if necessary) and bake until golden brown for 35-40 minutes (rotate the baking sheet for even baking halfway through).

5. Remove from the oven and allow to cool fully before melding with cranberries or dried

and raisins

6. To preserve additional crispiness, store in airtight containers in the fridge.

3.10 Whole Grain Cottage Cheese Pancakes

YIELD: 4 servings

Ingredients

- 1 cup oat flour
- 2 tbsp teff flour

- 1 tbsp baking powder
- 3 eggs
- 4 tsp canola oil
- 1-pint blueberries
- 1/2 cup sorghum flour
- 1/2 tsp salt
- 3 1/2 tsp sugar
- 1/2 tsp flax meal
- 1/2 tsp vanilla extract
- 1/2 cup maple syrup
- 1/3 cup plus 1 tbsp tapioca starch
- 1/3 cup cottage cheese
- 3/4 cup buttermilk
- 1 tsp lemon juice
- 3 tbsp water
- pinch of salt

Directions:

1. In a wide mixing bowl, combine all of your dried ingredients and stir to combine evenly.

2. In a separate container, mix all of your wet ingredients.

3. Create a well in the center of your dry ingredients and start pouring in the wet ingredients slowly, around a quarter cup at a time. This act will ensure that while whisking, no lumps form.

4. When a smooth batter appears, start to add the wet ingredients to the flour foundation. When you preheat your grill pan, let the butter for 15 minutes at rest.

5. Make a warm maple blueberry compote when the grill heats up. In a small pot, combine the blueberries, maple syrup, water, lemon juice, and salt pinch. For blending, whisk uniformly.

6. Heat the pot gently on low heat till the blueberries begin to pop, and their natural juices are

released. Put back, keep it warm.

7. Lightly oil the grill pan using the nonstick spray or use a limited volume of neutral-flavored oil until the grill pan is preheated to a medium-high temperature.

8. Scoop the batter on to the grill pan, and make sure that the griddle is not overcrowded.

9. Enable the pancakes to bake repeatedly until the sides look dry without cracking, and bubbles come to the top. This act should take about two minutes.

10. Turn the pancakes over and cook for another two minutes on the other side.

11. Keep warm or serve with the warm maple-blueberry compote immediately.

3.11 Very Berry Muesli

YIELD: 4 Servings

Ingredients

- Salt (Pinch)
- 1/4 cup toasted walnuts (chopped)
- 1/2 cup blueberries (frozen)
- 1/2 cup of dried fruit such as try raisins, dates and apricots
- 1/2 cup apple (chopped)
- 1/2 cup milk (1%)
- 1 cup of raw old-fashioned rolled oats
- 1 cup of fruit yogurt

Directions

1. Mix the oatmeal, milk, yogurt and salt in a medium dish.

2. For 6-12 hours, cover and refrigerate.

3. Gently mix and add dried and fresh berries.

4. In little bowls, serve spoonful of muesli. Sprinkle with chopped nuts for each meal.

5. Leftovers can be refrigerated within 2-3 hours.

3.12 Red Pepper, Kale, and Cheddar Frittata

YIELD: 6-8 SERVINGS

Ingredients

- 5 oz spinach and baby kale
- 3/4 cup of Milk
- 12 eggs
- 1/4 tablespoon salt
- 1/4 tablespoon pepper
- 1/3 cup sliced scallions
- 1 tablespoon olive oil
- 1 red pepper (diced)
- 1 cup cheddar cheese (sharp shredded)

Directions

1. Preheat the oven to 375 degrees Fahrenheit.

2. Spray with olive oil or nonstick spray on an 8 1/2-inch or 12-inch glass or casserole dish.

3. In a large frying pan, heat the oil. Stir in the red peppers and simmer until tender. Apply the kale and Spinach, stirring regularly or around 3 minutes before the greens are wilted.

4. Move the peppers and greens, scattered thinly to the bowl. Add the sliced scallions.

5. Consolidate the salt, milk, and pepper with the eggs. Over the pan, add the egg mixture. Sprinkle the end of the cheese.

6. Bake for 35-40 minutes, or when the mixture is perfectly set and lightly browned. Place under the broiler for just an additional 1 to 3 minutes to add the color and check thoroughly to ensure that the top does not burn. Until cutting, let it cool for about 5 minutes.

7. Serve it warm, or refrigerate throughout the week for a simple breakfast. Reheat the microwave for 1-2 minutes.

3.13 Veggie Quiche Muffins

YIELD: 12 Servings

Ingredients

- 4 eggs
- 3⁄4 cup of shredded cheddar cheese (low-fat)
- 2 cups milk (nonfat or 1%)
- 1⁄2 teaspoon salt
- 1⁄2 teaspoon pepper
- 1 teaspoon of Italian seasoning (or dried leaf basil & oregano)
- 1 cup tomatoes (diced)
- 1 cup green onion or onion (chopped)
- 1 cup broccoli (chopped)
- 1 cup baking mix (intended for pancakes or biscuits)

Directions:

1. Heat the oven to 375 °F. Lightly spray the12 muffin cups or oil them.

2. Sprinkle the muffin cups with cheese, broccoli, onions and tomatoes.

3. In a pan, put the rest of the ingredients and beat until smooth. In muffin cups, spill the egg mixture over the other ingredients.

4. Bake for 35-40 minutes, until the golden brown or the knife inserted in the middle comes out clean. Cool for five minutes.

5. Leftovers should be refrigerated within 2 hours.

3.14 Sweet Millet Congee

YIELD: 8 Servings

Ingredients

- 1⁄4 cup honey
- 1 cup of hulled millet

- 1 cup peeled and diced sweet potato
- 1 medium diced with skin apple
- 1 teaspoon of ground cinnamon
- 2 tablespoons of brown sugar
- 2 teaspoons of minced ginger (optional)
- 5 cups of water
- 8 bacon's strips

Directions:

1. Cook the bacon in a skillet until it becomes crispy, at medium-high heat. To eliminate extra fat, remove it from the pan and blot it with a paper towel. Crumble the bacon strips until it becomes cooled, and set aside.

2. Rinse the millet and drain it.

3. In a deep bath, mix the millet, water, ginger, cinnamon, sweet potato, and brown sugar. Ring to a simmering, reduce heat to low and boil until water evaporates (approximately 1 hour) and stirring regularly.

4. If the millet has been baked, remove the pot from the heat and add crumbles of apple, honey and bacon.

5. Method of slow cooking: Lessen the 1 cup water and cook 2 to 21⁄2 hours on high.

3.15 Turkey Sausage and Mushroom Strata

YIELD: 12 Servings

Ingredients

- ½ cup green onion (chopped)
- ½ teaspoon of paprika
- 1 cup mushrooms (sliced)
- 1-1/2 cup of 4 ounces cheddar cheese (reduced-fat shredded sharp)
- 12 ounces of egg's substitute

- 12 ounces of turkey sausage (can be frozen section)
- 2 cups milk (fat-free)
- 2 tablespoons parmesan cheese (grated)
- 3 large eggs
- 8 ounces of wheat ciabatta bread (1" cubes)
- Fresh ground pepper for taste

Directions

1. Preheat the oven to 400 degrees Fahrenheit.

2. On a baking sheet, place cubes of bread. Bake for 8 minutes at 400 °F or until it becomes toasted.

3. Over the medium-high flame, heat a medium skillet. Add the sausage to the pan; cook for just 7 minutes and stirring to crumble or until browned.

4. Add the milk, eggs, egg substitute, cheese, parmesan cheese, salt, paprika, and pepper with a whisk in a big cup.

5. Add the sausage bread, mushrooms and scallions, and toss to cover the bread well. Do spoon mixing in a 13*9-inch baking pan. Cover it and refrigerate for 8 hours or overnight.

6. Preheat the furnace to 27 °F.

7. Uncover the casserole. Bake for 50 minutes at 350 °F or until lightly browned. Split into 12 pieces and serve instantly.

3.16 Summer Breakfast Quinoa Bowls

YIELD**:** 2 Servings

Ingredients

- ¾ + 2/3 cup milk (low-fat)
- 2 teaspoons of honey
- 2 teaspoons of brown sugar
- 14 blueberries
- 12 raspberries

- 1/3 cup well-rinsed uncooked quinoa
- 1/2 teaspoon of vanilla extract
- 1 small sliced peach

Directions:

1. In a saucepan, combine quinoa and 2/3 cup milk, vanilla and brown sugar.

2. Cook on medium heat and bring to boil for five minutes. Reduce heat to low and cover it. Cook for 15 to 20 minutes, or until easily fluffs with a fork.

3. Meanwhile, heat a grill pan and spray with oil. Grill the peaches to bring out their sweetness 2 to 3 minutes and set aside. Warm the remaining milk in the microwave.

4. Divide the cooked quinoa between 2 bowls, then pour in warmed milk. Top with peaches, raspberries and blueberries and drizzle each with 1 teaspoon of honey.

3.17 Strawberry Breakfast Sandwich (Halves)

YIELD: 8 Servings

Ingredients

- 1 tablespoon of honey
- 1 teaspoon of grated Lemon zest
- 2 cups 10-ounces strawberries (sliced)
- 4 split and toasted English muffins
- 8-ounces Neufchatel cheese/low-fat softened cream cheese

Directions:

1. In a food processor, process the honey, cheese and zest until they become fully mixed. You can mix in a bowl with a wooden spoon.

2. Unfurl the 1 tablespoon of cheese mixture on the cut side of 1 muffin half and top with 1 quarter cup of strawberries.

3. Perform the same procedure with the remaining ingredients to make eight half-sandwiches.

3.18 Spinach, Mushroom, and Feta Cheese Scramble

YIELD: 1 Serving

Ingredients

- ½ cup fresh sliced mushrooms
- 1 cup fresh chopped Spinach
- 2 egg whites & 1 whole egg
- 2 tablespoons of feta cheese
- Cooking spray
- Pepper for taste

Directions:

1. On medium fire, heat an 8-inch nonstick sauté tray. Using cooking spray to spray and include mushrooms and Spinach.

2. Sauté the Spinach and mushrooms for 2-3 minutes or before the spinach wilts.

3. If needed, whisk the egg and egg whites into a bowl of feta cheese and pepper. Pour the egg mixture into the pan over the vegetables.

4. Continue to cook the eggs for another 3-4 minutes while stirring with a spatula or until the eggs are cooked completely.

3.19 Steel Cut Oat Blueberry Pancakes

YIELD: 10 Servings

Ingredients

- ½ cup + 2 tablespoons of agave nectar
- ½ cup vanilla flavor Greek yogurt
- ½ cup of steel-cut oats
- ½ teaspoon of baking powder
- 1 cup blueberries (frozen)
- 1 cup of Milk

- 1 cup of whole wheat flour
- 1 egg
- 1/8 teaspoon of sea salt
- 1-1/2 cups of water

Directions:

1. Bring water to boil in a medium pot and add salt and steel-cut oats. Reduce the heat to a low simmer and cook for about 10 minutes until the oats are tender. Remove from the heat.

2.Combine the whole wheat pastry flour, baking powder, egg, baking soda, milk and yogurt in a medium mixing dish. Mix it to shapes a batter. Gently fold in the cooked oats and blueberries.

3. Heat a medium-heated grill rack or nonstick skillet and spray with cooking oil. Spoon a quarter cup of batter on the surface and cook until the pancakes start bubbling and are mildly brown. If necessary, operating in batches around 2-3 minutes per hand.

4. Garnish with around one tablespoon agave for each pancake

3.20 Cabbage And Dal Paratha

YIELD: 4 Servings

Ingredients

For Dough

- ½ cup of oats flour and ½ cup wheat flour
- ¼ tablespoon salt

For Stuffing

- ¼ cup of finely chopped mint leaves
- ¼ cup of soaked & boiled moong dal
- ¼ cup of finely chopped onions
- ¾ cup of finely chopped cabbage
- 1 pinch of turmeric powder
- 1 tablespoon fennel seeds

- 1 tablespoon grated ginger
- 1 tablespoon oil
- 1/8 tablespoon salt
- 2 tablespoons dry mango powder
- 2 tablespoon finely chopped green chilies

Directions:

For Dough

1. In a cup, combine the wheat flour, oatmeal and salt.

2. Add sufficient water to make a moist pastry.

3. For 3-4 minutes, knead the mixture very well and place it aside.

For Stuffing

1. Heat the oil in the pan first, then cook the fennel seeds.

2. Put the onions in sauté until golden brown.

3. Then add green chilies and cabbage and cook for a minute on a medium flame.

4. Put the mint leaves, dried mango powder, turmeric, and 1 tbsp of water to the moong dal. Mix and cook over a medium flame for 2 minutes.

5. Divide the mixture into five equal parts.

Making Of Paratha

1. Create five equal pieces of the dough

2. Roll the dough out in a circle,

3. In the middle of the rolled circle, put a part of the stuffing.

4. Start to get both sides together in the middle. Tightly seal it

5. By using a rolling pin, roll the stuffed dough into a circle again (for fast-rolling, sprinkle the wheat flour on a rolling base)

6. Use a preheated pan to cook both sides of the paratha until golden brown. Use the 1/4 tsp of oil.

7. Ready to feed, piping hot and nutrient-filled cabbage and dal paratha. Serve along with tomato

chutney or mint.

3.21 Red Velvet Pancakes with Cream Cheese Topping

YIELD: 5 Servings

Ingredients

Cream Cheese Topping:

- 1 tablespoon milk (fat-free)
- 2 ounces 1/3 cream cheese (less fat)
- 3 tablespoons honey
- 3 tablespoons of plain yogurt (fat-free)

Pancakes:

- 2 ¼ teaspoons of baking powder
- 1 teaspoon vanilla
- 1 large egg
- 2 tablespoons + 1 cup milk (fat-free)
- ½ teaspoon food coloring (red paste)
- ½ tablespoon cocoa powder (unsweetened)
- ½ cup of whole wheat flour
- ½ cup all-purpose flour (unbleached)
- ¼ teaspoon of salt
- ¼ cup of sugar

Directions:

1. Mix and set aside the cream cheese coating ingredients.
2. In a large dish, combine the flour, baking powder, chocolate powder, sugar, and salt.
3. Dissolve the food coloring with the milk in another one; whisk in the egg and vanilla.
4. Take note not to overmix the wet and dry products until there are no longer dry spots.

5. On a medium-low fire, heat a large nonstick griddle pan. Spray lightly with oil to cover when wet, and spill 1⁄4 cup of the pancake batter into the pan.

6. Flip the pancakes as long as the pancake begins to bubble, and the edges start to settle. Repeat for the remaining batter.

7. Place 2 pancakes on each plate to eat, then finish with approximately 2-1⁄2 tablespoons of cream cheese topping.

3.22 Scrambled Eggs with Spinach

YIELD: 1 serving

Ingredients

- 2 Eggs
- 1 medium tomato (chopped)
- ½ teaspoon of cayenne pepper
- ½ teaspoon of fresh basil or cilantro or parsley
- ¼ cup of Swiss cheese
- 1 large handful of Spinach chopped

Directions:

1. Mix the chickens, basil and cayenne pepper in a large bowl. To beat until frothy, use a rotational beater or wire whisk.
2. Pour into a ready-made skillet. Start softly yet constantly stirring eggs immediately with a plastic or wooden spatula until the mixture resembles small fragments of fried egg covered by liquid egg. Add the tomatoes and Spinach.
3. Cook for an additional 30 to 60 seconds or until the egg is fixed but glossy.
4. Sprinkle with cheese (swiss) and new ground pepper.
5. Cover it with parsley.
6. Raise and fold one side of the omelet partly over the filling, using a spatula.
7. On a warm platter, arrange the remaining Spinach.

3.23 Tofu and Mushroom Scramble

YIELD: 3 servings

Ingredients

- A little lemon/lime juice
- ½ Avocado (ripe)
- 1 package of pressed tofu or extra-firm (crumbled)
- 1/2 diced red pepper
- 1/2 tablespoon of cumin, chili powder, garlic powder & chia seeds, pepper
- 1/4 cup of grated carrot
- 1/4 cup of diced red onion
- 2 cloves of garlic
- 2 Spring Onions (finely chopped)
- 4 large sliced white mushrooms
- Turmeric mixed with 3 tablespoons of water

Directions:

1. Over medium fire, heat a nonstick pan.
2. Add the garlic, red pepper, red onion, mushrooms and grated carrot and simmer for around 6 to 7 minutes before the onions and mushrooms start to soften.
3. When required, add a little water.
4. To the pan, add the crumbled tofu and spice mixture.
5. Stir well to mix it all up and fry before the tofu is cooked up.
6. Serve in a cup and finish with sliced avocado and scatter with spring onions and lemon or lime juice.

3.24 MUSHROOM and SAUSAGE QUICHE

YIELD: 2 servings

Ingredients

- ¼ cup of Swiss Cheese (grated)
- ¼ cup of sliced scallions
- ½ teaspoon of ground black pepper
- 1 cup of milk (1%)
- 1 teaspoon olive oil
- 3 egg whites
- 5 eggs
- 6 oz mushrooms
- 8 oz of turkey breakfast sausage with removed casing (cut into small pieces)

Directions:

1. Over medium-high heat, heat a large nonstick skillet. Add the sausage and cook for 6 to 8 minutes, until golden brown. Move it to a bowl for cooling.
2. To the pan, add oil. Add the mushrooms and cook, constantly stirring for 5 to 7 minutes, until golden brown. Transfer the mushrooms to the sausage bowl.
3. Leave for 5 minutes to cool. Stir in the scallions, pepper and cheese.
4. In a medium dish, whisk together the eggs, egg whites, and milk. Divide the egg mixture equally between the muffin cups that have been packed. Sprinkle the sausage mixture with a heaping tablespoon into each cup.
5. Place the rack in the middle of the oven; preheat to 325 °F. Kindly coat a nonstick muffin pan with cooking oil.
6. Bake until the tops tend to brown, for 25 minutes. Let it cool for 5 minutes on a wire rack. On top of the pan, place a plate, flip it over, and switch the quiches out off the rack. Turn upright and let it cool.

3.25 Turmeric Milk

YIELD: 1 serving

Ingredients

- ½ teaspoon of turmeric powder
- ½ teaspoon of vanilla extract
- 1 tablespoon coconut oil
- 2 Cups of warm almond milk

Directions:

Blend or whisk until frothy and enjoy.

3.26 Poached Eggs with Avocado and Balsamic Tomatoes

YIELD: 2 servings

Ingredients

- 1 tablespoon of mixed Italian herbs or thyme
- 2 avocados
- 2 tablespoons of balsamic vinegar
- 2 tablespoons of olive oil
- per person 2 to 3 eggs
- 8 -10 tomatoes

Directions:

1. Put a pot of water to a boil (use sufficient water while the eggs are on the bottom to coat them). Directly smash the eggs into the boiling water, turn the heat down to mild for 2 minutes and then extract the product.
2. Chop up some tomatoes and cut the avocado while the eggs are frying. Use a spatula to separate the eggs from the water until the eggs are set.
3. Sprinkle with the Italian herbs, fresh herbs, and pepper; eat with fresh heirloom tomatoes, or roast with some balsamic vinegar if you have time.

3.27 Guacamole Deviled Eggs

YIELD: 3 servings

Ingredients

- 1 tablespoon of chives or green onion
- 1 tablespoon of Cilantro
- 1 tablespoon of Lime
- 1 tablespoon of Sour cream
- 1/2 chili pepper (jalapeno)
- 2 Avocados (ripe)
- 6 eggs (Hard Boiled) without shell and cut partially

Directions:

Add the ingredients in a bowl and mash with a yellow portion of an egg, slice the avocados, cut the pit and scoop the fruit out into a dish.

3.28 Pineapple Protein Smoothie

YIELD: 2 servings

Ingredients

- 2 tablespoon almond butter
- 2 dates (pitted)
- 2 tablespoon ground turmeric
- 1/2 cup of ice
- 3/4 cup of Milk
- 3/4 cup of pineapple chunks
- 3/4 cup of rinsed and drained canned chickpeas

Directions:

Mix all the ingredients until smooth.

3.29 Mixed Vegetable Thoran

YIELD: 2 servings

Ingredients

- ¼ cup of green peas
- ¼ tablespoon urad dal
- ½ cup of finely chopped carrots
- ½ cup of finely chopped French beans
- ½ cup of chopped onions
- ½ tablespoon chili powder
- ½ tablespoon mustard seeds
- ½ tablespoon roasted cumin seeds
- 1 tablespoon oil
- 1/8 tablespoon salt
- 2 Kashmiri red chilies
- 2 tablespoons crushed garlic

Directions:

1. Heat the oil and place the mustard seeds in a pan.

2. Put urad dal, red chilies and garlic and sauté on a medium flame for 1 min until the seeds start to crackle.

3. Then add onions, carrots, French beans, salt & peas and sauté on a medium flame for 2 minutes again.

4. Then apply 2 teaspoons of water and mix them well.

5. Cover the pan with a lid and cook the mixture for 5-6 minutes over medium heat. stir occasionally.

6. Then add chili powder, ground cumin seeds and mix well. On a medium flame, cook this mixture for 1 minute. Stir occasionally

7. Your tasty and high in health and low salt and the vegetable dish is ready to eat. Serve with Bajra/Jowar Rotis and even better with wheat Rotis (both are rich in potassium, which is important for lowering blood pressure).

Chapter 4 - Lunch Recipes

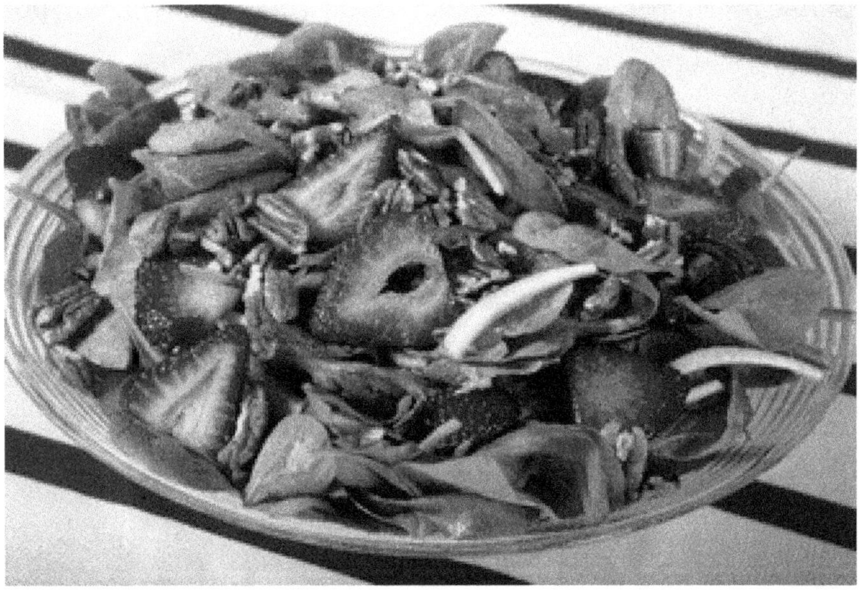

4.1 Quinoa Meatless Balls

YIELD: 24 servings

Ingredients

- 1 3/4 cup of grain bread crumbs
- 1 onion
- 1 tablespoon of olive oil (extra virgin)
- 1/2 tablespoon sea salt
- 1/3 cup of chives
- 1/3 cup of parmesan cheese
- 2 1/2 cup of cooked quinoa
- 3 cloves of garlic
- 4 eggs

Directions:

1. In a bowl, add all the ingredients and mix.
2. Mix Mold into meatballs.

3. The skillet is dipped with olive oil (extra virgin).

4. Brown the meatballs for 10 minutes in a pan.

4.2 Quesadillas with Cilantro Yogurt Dip

YIELD: 4 Servings

Ingredients

- ½ finely chopped bell pepper
- ½ cup corn kernels
- ½ finely minced jalapeno pepper (optional)
- 1 cup of beans (black or pinto)
- 1 cup of low-fat cheese (shredded)
- 1 cup plain yogurt (nonfat)
- 1 medium carrot (shredded)
- 2 tablespoons cilantro (chopped)
- 2 Tablespoons cilantro (finely chopped)
- 6 corn tortillas (soft)
- Cilantro yogurt dip
- ½ of a lime Juice

Directions:

1. Over the low heat, preheat a large skillet.

2. Place 3 tortillas in rows. Divide the tortillas on cheese, rice, corn, cilantro, sliced carrots, and peppers.

3. With a second tortilla, cover each one.

4. Put a tortilla on the dry skillet and heat for about 3 minutes before the cheese melts, and the tortilla is somewhat golden.

5. Flip and cook until golden from the other side, around 1 minute.

6. Mix the nonfat cream, lime juice and cilantro in a shallow dish.

4.3 Cauliflower Steak

YIELD: 2 SERVINGS

Ingredients

- ½ tablespoon of salt & pepper
- 1 head cauliflower
- 1 sprig chopped & stemmed thyme (fresh)
- 1 tablespoon chopped fresh rosemary
- 2 tablespoon olive oil (extra virgin)
- 3 minced cloves garlic
- 3 chopped sage leaves
- black pepper (fresh ground)

Directions:

1. Preheat to 400 °F in your oven. Remove the cauliflower leaves from the end of the stem, leaving the heart intact. Place the center side of the cauliflower down on a cutting board. Slice the cauliflower into four steaks from the middle of the cauliflower by using a large knife. Every steak should have a thickness of around a half-inch.

2. Put parchment paper on the baking sheet and use a teaspoon of olive oil to the top. On the baking dish, arrange the cauliflower steaks together with some of the split florets.

3. Combine most olive oil, chopped garlic, salt, pepper, and herbs in a separate dish. With this combination, spray the cauliflower slices evenly on both sides, but make sure the oil and herbs protect all the crevices.

4. Roast for 20 minutes in the oven. Flip the cauliflower and bake until golden brown and cooked through for another 10 minutes.

5. Remove from the oven when the cauliflower steaks are cooked, and transfer to the individual serving plates. Season with the fresh ground black pepper in a generous amount.

4.4 Sunshine Wrap

YIELD: 4 Servings

Ingredients

- ¼ cup minced onion
- ¼ teaspoon of black pepper
- ¼ teaspoon of garlic powder
- ½ cup diced celery
- 1 large wheat tortilla (whole)
- 1 teaspoon of soy sauce
- 2 tablespoons of mayonnaise
- 2/3 cup of canned mandarin oranges (drained)
- 4 large washed & patted dry lettuce leaves
- 8 oz chicken breast piece (one large)

Directions:

1. In a nonstick pan, cook chicken breast on medium-high heat until the internal temperature hits the 165°F. When the chicken has cooled enough to handle, cut into ½ inch cubes.

2. In a medium-sized bowl, mix the onions, oranges, chicken and celery. Add mayonnaise, garlic, pepper and soy sauce. Meld gently until chicken mixture is uniformly coated.

3. Put the tortilla on a neat cutting board or open plate. With a sharp knife or clean kitchen scissors, cut the tortilla into four quarters. Set 1 lettuce leaf on each tortilla quarter, trimming the leaf to

hang over the tortilla.

4. Put one-fourth part of the chicken mixture in the center of every lettuce leaf. Roll up the tortillas

into a cone shape, with the two edges getting together and the arched edge creating the cone's opening. Eat like a sandwich wrap.

5. Refrigerate leftovers within 2 hours.

7. Cut each quesadilla into 4 wedges (12 wedges total) and serve 3 wedges per person with about ¼ cup of the dip.

8. Refrigerate leftovers within 2 hours.

4.5 Southwest Style Rice Bowl

YIELD: 2 Servings

Ingredients

- 4 tablespoons of salsa
- 2 tablespoons of shredded cheese
- 2 tablespoons of sour cream (low fat)
- 1 teaspoon of vegetable oil
- 1 cup chopped or shredded cooked meat
- 1 cup brown rice (cooked)
- 1 cup vegetable mixture - onion bell peppers, zucchini, corn and tomato (chopped).

Directions:

1. Heat up the oil in a medium skillet over medium-high heat (in an electric skillet at 350 degrees Fahrenheit). Add the vegetables and cook for 3-5 minutes or until the vegetables are crisp and tender.

2. On the skillet, add cooked beef, tofu or beans and cooked rice and fire.

3. Split the rice mixture into two containers. Cover with cheese, sour cream & salsa and serve it warm.

4. Leftovers should be refrigerated within 2 hours.

4.6 Southwestern Black Bean Cakes with Guacamole

YIELD: 4 Servings

Ingredients

- ½ medium seeded & peeled avocado
- 1 (15-ounce) rinsed & drained low sodium black beans
- 1 (7-ounce) chipotle peppers (in adobo sauce)
- 1 large egg
- 1 plum tomato (small)

- 1 tablespoon of lime juice
- 1 teaspoon of ground cumin
- 2 cloves of garlic
- 2 slices of whole wheat bread (torn)
- 3 tablespoons of fresh cilantro

Directions:

1. In a food processor bowl or blender, put the broken bread. Cover and process or mix until coarse crumbs imitate the bread. Place the crumbs in a big bowl and set them aside.

2. Using cilantro and garlic to process or combine until finely chopped. Add 1 or 2 teaspoons of adobo sauce, rice, 1 chipotle pepper, and cumin. The mixture starts to pull away from the sides using on/off pulses to process or combine until the beans are coarsely sliced.

3. In a cup, add the mixture to the bread crumbs. Add the egg and mix thoroughly.

4. Shape the mixture into four 1/2-inch-thick patties. Grill these on a lightly oil uncovered grill rack directly on medium heat for about 8 to 10 minutes or until the patties are heated. Rotate once.

5. Similarly, to mash avocado in small cups. Stir in the lime juice. Season with salt and pepper. Serve with guacamole and tomato patties.

4.7 Pesto & Mozzarella Stuffed Portobello Mushroom Caps

YIELD: 1 Serving

Ingredients

- ¼ cup of shredded mozzarella cheese (low-fat)
- 1 small diced Roma tomato
- 2 mushroom caps (portobello)
- 2 tablespoons of pesto

Directions:

1. Clean the mushrooms by using a dry or moist rag. By twisting softly, remove the roots.

2. Divide the pesto uniformly between the 2 caps of the mushroom.

3. Cover with chopped and shredded tomatoes and cheese.

4. Bake in the oven at 400 °F for 15 minutes.

4.8 Mayo-less Tuna Salad

YIELD: 2 Servings

Ingredients

- black pepper
- 5 oz. light tuna in water (drained)
- 2 cups of arugula
- 1 tablespoon of red wine vinegar
- 1 tablespoon of shaved parmesan cheese (fresh)
- 1 tablespoon of olive oil (extra virgin)
- 1 cup of cooked pasta from 2 oz dry
- ¼ cup green onion tops (chopped)

Directions:

1. Toss the tuna with the oil, onion, vinegar, cooked pasta and arugula in a large bowl.

2. On two plates, divide and top with pepper and Parmesan.

3. Serve Instantly.

4.9 Washington Apple Turkey Gyro

YIELD: 6 Servings

Ingredients

- ½ cup of plain yogurt (low fat/fat-free)
- ½ pound cooked chicken breast/turkey (cut into thin strips)
- 1 cored apple, if possible Golden Delicious; (finely chopped or sliced),
- 1 cup onion (sliced)
- 1 cup of sweet green pepper (thinly sliced)

- 1 cup of sweet red pepper (thinly sliced)
- 1 tablespoon of vegetable oil
- 2 tablespoons of lemon juice
- 6 warmed pocket pita bread (whole wheat)

Directions:

1. Heat the oil in a large skillet over medium heat. Place the onion, peppers and lemon juice in the mixture and cook until tender. Mix in the apple turkey and cook until the turkey is heated. Simply remove from the heat.

2. Cover with some of the mixtures for each pita; drizzle with the yogurt. Serve it warm.

4.10 Fresh Shrimp Spring Rolls

YIELD: 6 Servings

Ingredients

- ½ medium cucumber (thinly sliced)
- ¾ cup cilantro (fresh)
- 1 ¼ pounds-20 ounces cooked shrimp (deveined & peeled)
- 1 cup shredded carrots
- 12 basil leaves
- 12 bibs of lettuce leaves
- 12 sheets of rice paper

Directions:

1. Clean the lettuce, basil, cilantro, carrots and cucumber, and make them ready.

2. For quick access, place all the vegetables and shrimp on the counter assembly-line style.

3. On a clean cutting board, put down a wet paper towel. Place one sheet of rice paper on a paper towel under warm water till it wets.

4. Layer 1 leaf of lettuce, 1 leaf of basil, 1 tablespoon of cilantro, cucumber and carrots on the rice paper that is nearest to you at the end. Begin gently rolling the rice paper over the vegetables like

a burrito.

5. Place around 4 shrimp on the rice paper while the vegetables are covered. Continue to fold up the rice paper like a burrito until it's all rolled up, and do not forget to tuck in the ends.

6. Repeat the process before you make all 12 rolls. Serve them immediately.

4.11 Pear, Turkey and Cheese Sandwich

YIELD: 2 Servings

Ingredients

- 1 USA pear, cored and thinly sliced
- 1/4 cup shredded low-fat mozzarella cheese
- 2 slices (1 oz. each) reduced-sodium cooked or smoked turkey
- 2 tsp Dijon-style mustard
- Coarsely ground pepper

Directions:

1. Spread 1 teaspoon of mustard on each slice of bread. Place each slice of bread with one slice of turkey. Arrange the turkey pear slices and sprinkle each with 2 tablespoons of cheese. Sprinkle pepper over it.

2. Broil for 2 to 3 minutes by keeping 4 to 6 inches away from the heat or until turkey and pears become heated and cheese melts. Slice each sandwich in half and serve open face.

4.12 Spinach, Mushroom and Mozzarella Wraps

YIELD: 2 Servings

Ingredients

- ¼ cup 1-ounce part-skim mozzarella cheese (shredded)
- ½ pound trimmed & steamed fresh spinach/arugula
- 1 plum diced tomato
- 1 tablespoon of olive oil
- 1 teaspoon of minced garlic

- 2 whole wheat of 8-inch tortillas
- 8 oz. fresh sliced mushrooms (approximately 2 ½ cups)

Directions:

1. Preheat the furnace to 350 °F. Heat 1 tablespoon olive oil over high heat in a saucepan. Add the single piece of garlic and mushrooms. Be vigilant as they turn red-brown, then turn and sauté until the second side becomes the same.

2. Spread layers of lettuce, mozzarella, cooked mushrooms and onion on each tortilla. Roll up and put in a finely oiled baking bowl, seam-side down. Bake until the cheese is melted and warm for about 10 minutes.

3. Slice each tortilla into quarters crosswise. Serve as desired at warm or room temperature.

4.13 Heartfelt Tuna Melt

YIELD: 4 Servings

Ingredients

- Salt & black pepper for taste
- 6 ounces drained white tuna (packed in water)
- 3 ounces grated Cheddar cheese (reduced-fat)
- 2 whole-wheat split English muffins
- 1/4 cup Russian (low fat) or Island salad dressing
- 1/4 cup onion (chopped)
- 1/3 cup celery (chopped)

Directions:

1. Preheat the broiler.

2. Put the salmon, celery, salad dressing and onion together. season with salt and pepper.

3. Toast half the English muffin. On the baking sheet, put split-side-up and cover each one with 1/4 of the tuna mixture. Broil for 2-3 minutes or until completely cooked.

4. Top with the cheese and return to the broiler for about 1 minute before the cheese is melted.

4.14 Apple-Swiss Panini

YIELD: 4 Servings

Ingredients

- ¼ cup of honey mustard (nonfat)
- 1 cup of arugula leaves
- 2 thinly sliced crisp apples,
- 6 ounces thinly sliced Swiss cheese (low-fat)
- 8 slices of whole-grain bread
- Cooking spray

Directions:

1. On medium-heat, Preheat the panini press. Use just a nonstick skillet if you don't have a panini press.

2. Apply the honey mustard, gently and uniformly over each bread slice. Layer four slices of bread with apple slices, butter, and arugula leaves. Top each one with the remaining slices of bread.

3. Lightly coat the cooking spray with the panini press. Grill every sandwich for about 3 to 5 mins or until it is melted with cheese and toasted with bread. Remove from the pan before serving and let it to cool slightly.

4.15 California Grilled Veggie Sandwich

YIELD: 4 Servings

Ingredients

- ½ cup crumbled feta cheese (reduced-fat)
- 1 cup of sliced red bell peppers
- 1 sliced red onion
- 1 sliced small yellow squash
- 1 small sliced zucchini
- 1 tablespoon of lemon juice

- 1/8 cup of olive oil
- 2 slices of focaccia bread
- 3 cloves garlic (minced)
- 3 tablespoons of light mayonnaise

Directions:

1. Meld the mayonnaise, minced garlic, and lemon juice in a cup. Keep it in the refrigerator.

2. Preheat the grill to a high degree.

3. Brush the vegetables with olive oil. Brush the barbecue grill with oil. Place the bell peppers and zucchini nearest to the center of the grill and place bits of onion and squash around them. Cook for 3 minutes, turn and cook for 3 more minutes. It will take much longer for the peppers. Remove and set aside from the barbecue.

4. On the crust's cut sides, scatter some of the mayonnaise mixtures; sprinkle all with the feta cheese. Put on the grill in cheese side up position, and cover for 2 to 3 min with the lid. Carefully watch it so as not to burn the bottoms.

5. Take the bread from the grill and layer the vegetables with it. Enjoy the open-faced grilled sandwiches.

4.16 Terrific Tortellini Salad

YIELD: 8 main-dish Servings

Ingredients

- Milk (optional)
- 3 cups of broccoli florets
- 1/4 cup green onions (sliced)
- 1/2 cup bottled ranch salad dressing (reduced-fat)
- 1 large tomato (chopped)
- 1 cup of fresh pea pods (halved)
- 1 cup of crinkle-cut/sliced carrots - 2 medium
- 1 9-ounce package of refrigerated light cheese tortellini/ravioli

Directions:

1. Cook the pasta according to product instructions in a large saucepan. During the last 3 minutes of preparation, add the broccoli and carrots. Drain it. Rinse with some cold water. Again drain it.

2. Mix the cooked pasta mixture and green onions in a large bowl; sprinkle with dressing. To coat, toss softly. For 2 to 24 hours, cover it and then cool.

3. Stir the tomato and pea pods gently into the pasta mixture before eating. To moisten, stir in a little milk if necessary. For serving, make eight main-dishes.

4.17 Tuscan-Style Tuna Salad

YIELD: 4 (1 cup each) Servings

Ingredients

- 1 15-ounce can of small white beans like cannellini/great northern (rinsed)
- 1/4 teaspoon salt
- 10 cherry tomatoes (quartered)
- 2 6-ounce cans of chunk light tuna (drained)
- 2 tablespoons of olive oil (extra-virgin)
- 2 tablespoons of lemon juice
- 4 scallions (trimmed & sliced)
- Freshly ground pepper for taste

Directions:

1. In a medium dish, combine the fish, beans, onions, oil, scallions, lemon juice, pepper, and salt.
2. Stir it slowly. Refrigerate until it is ready.

4.18 Strawberry, Melon & Avocado Salad

YIELD: 4 Servings

Ingredients

- 1 1/2 cups sliced hulled strawberries

- 1 small avocado 4-5 ounces (peeled up, pitted and cut into 16 slices)
- 1/4 cup honey
- 1/4 teaspoon ground pepper (fresh)
- 16 slices of about 1/2 small cantaloupe (thin & rind removed)
- 2 tablespoons fresh mint (finely chopped)
- 2 tablespoons of sherry vinegar/red-wine vinegar
- 2 teaspoons toasted sesame seeds
- 4 cups of baby spinach
- Pinch of salt

Directions:

1. In a small cup, whisk the honey, mint, vinegar, pepper and salt.

2. Divide the Spinach into 4 plates of lettuce. On top of the Spinach, place alternating pieces of cantaloupe and avocado. Top the strawberries for each salad, sprinkle with dressing and scatter with the sesame seeds.

4.19 Roast Chicken Dal

YIELD: 4 (1 1/2 cups each) Servings

Ingredients

- 1 1/2 teaspoons of canola oil
- 1 14-ounce canned tomatoes (diced & preferably fire-roasted)
- 1 15-ounce lentil Can (rinsed) or 2 cups of cooked lentils
- 1 2-pound of roasted chicken with discarded skin, meat separated from bones & diced (4 cups)
- 1 small onion (minced)
- 1/4 cup plain yogurt (low-fat)
- 1/4 teaspoon salt for taste
- 2 teaspoons of curry powder

Directions:

1. Heat oil over medium to high heat heavy saucepan. Include the onion and fry, stirring for 3 to 4 minutes, until tender but not browned.
2. Add the curry powder and simmer for 20 to 30 seconds, stirring until mixed with the onion and deep aromatics.
3. Whisk in lentils, tomatoes, salt and chicken and cook until it is heated fully, stirring regularly.
4. Turn off the heat and apply the yogurt, and stir. Serve it instantly.

4.20 Spaghetti Squash with Chunky Tomato Sauce

YIELD: 6 Servings

Ingredients

- 1 pound of lean ground beef
- 2 cloves of minced garlic
- 2 tablespoons of tomato paste
- 1 recipe Cooked Spaghetti Squash
- Small & fresh basil leaves
- 1 14 1/2-ounce Canned tomatoes (diced & undrained)
- 1/2 cup 1 medium onion (chopped)
- 1/2 cup 1 small green sweet pepper (chopped)
- 1-1/2 teaspoons crushed Italian seasoning (dried)
- 1/4 cup 1-ounce Parmesan cheese (shredded)
- 1 8-ounce tomato sauce Can
- 1/8 teaspoon of black pepper

Directions:

1. Cook the ground beef, sweet pepper onion, and garlic in a wide saucepan until the meat is brown. Drain it. Add the diced and undrained tomatoes, black pepper tomato sauce, tomato paste, and Italian seasoning. Boil the sauce and minimize the heat. Simmer and uncovered for 15 minutes

and stir for some time.

2. Meanwhile, cooking of the Spaghetti Squash. Serve the sauce over squash. Sprinkle the cheese with Parmesan. Garnish with basil leaves if needed.

3. Cooked Spaghetti Squash: In many spots, a sharp knife pokes a 2-1/2 - 3-pound whole spaghetti squash. Put the squash in a microwave-safe baking dish. Microwave the uncovered for 10 to 15 minutes on 100 percent (high) capacity or until tender. Let wait for five minutes. Halve the thickness of the squash and cut the seeds. Shred and split the squash pulp into strands using two forks. Make 6 parts for serving.

Chapter 5 – Dinner

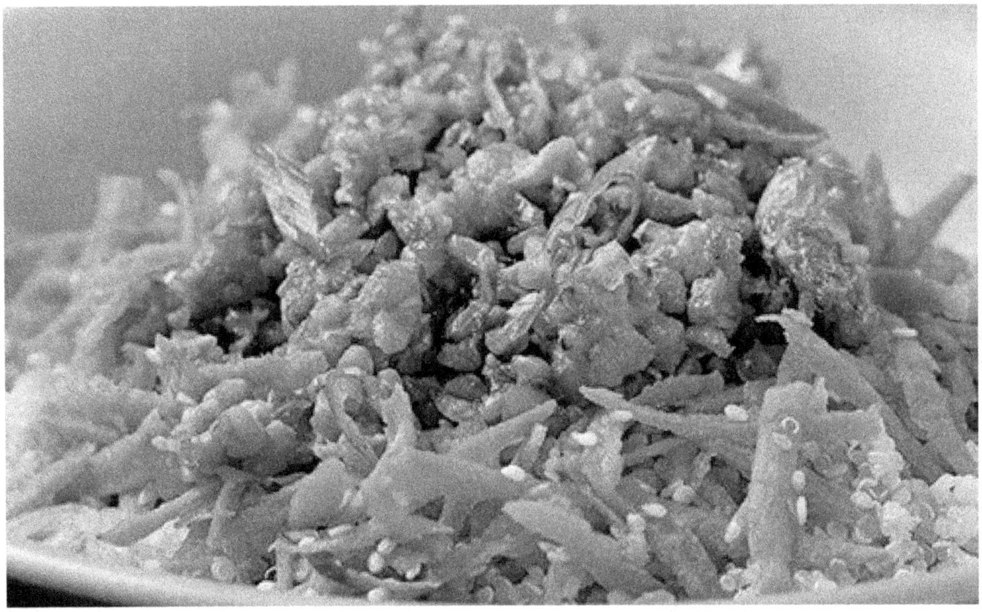

5.1 Meatier Meatloaf

YIELD: 6 servings

Ingredients

- 6 oz. of white mushrooms (trimmed & thinly sliced)
- 3/4 pepper
- 3 tablespoons with 1/2 cup chicken broth (low-sodium)
- 3 tablespoons of packed brown sugar
- 2 tablespoons of Dijon mustard
- 2 tablespoons of unsalted butter
- 2 tablespoons of soy sauce
- 2 large eggs
- 2 minced garlic cloves
- 1/4 cup of cider vinegar
- 1/3 cup fresh parsley (minced)
- 1/2 tablespoon of ground coriander

- 1/2 tablespoon of dried thyme
- 1/2 slice of white sandwich bread (split into 1" piece)
- 1/2 cup of ketchup
- 1 tablespoon of hot sauce
- 1 tablespoon of unflavored gelatin
- 1 tablespoon of tomato paste
- 1 onion (chopped & fine)
- 1-pound ground pork
- 1-pound lean ground beef (85%)

Directions:

1. For the meatloaf: Change the oven rack's center location and fire the oven to 350 degrees Fahrenheit. Fold heavy-duty aluminum foil into a 5-inch rectangle to form 9. Cover the foil in a rimmed baking sheet mounted on a wire shelf. Poke holes with a skewer (approximately 1/2 inch apart) in the foil. Spray the foil with a spray of vegetable oil.

2. In a 12-inch skillet over medium heat, melt the butter. Add the onion and mushrooms; fry and stirring regularly for 10 to 12 minutes, until the color is brown. Add the tomato paste and simmer for about 3 minutes and mix continuously, until browned. Reduce heat to low and add 3 tablespoons of broth and garlic. Cook to remove any browned pieces, scraping the plate's bottom until thickened, for around 1 minute. To cool, shift the mushroom mixture to a wide dish.

3. Whisk together the eggs, the remaining half a cup of broth, and the soy sauce in a bowl. Sprinkle the gelatin over the egg mixture and leave to rest for about 5 minutes until the gelatin softens.

4. Pulse the bread until finely ground in the food processor at 5 to 10 pulses. To bread-crumbs, add gelatin blend, cooled mushroom blend, mustard, parsley, thyme and pepper. And pulse them until the mushrooms are finely ground, around 10 pulses, scraping down the bowl as desired. Place the bread-crumb mixture in a wide dish. To fully blend, add pork and beef and meld with your hands.

5. Move the meat mixture to the rectangle foil and use wet hands to create a 9 by 5-inch loaf. Bake the meatloaf for 75 to 90 minutes until the heat reaches 155 to 160 degrees Fahrenheit. Take the

broiler from the oven and turn it on.

6. For the glaze: When the meatloaf is frying, put all the ingredients in a small saucepan over medium heat to boil. Cook and stirring regularly for about 5 minutes, until it becomes thick and syrupy.

7. Spread half of the glaze uniformly over the cooked meatloaf; put under the broiler and cook for around 2 minutes before the glaze bubbles and starts browning at the edges. Remove the meatloaf from the oven and cover thinly with the remaining glaze. Return to the broiler and cook for about 2 minutes longer before the glaze bursts again and starts to brown. Before slicing and serving, let the meatloaf cool for 20 minutes.

5.2 Salmon With Broccoli & Red Potatoes

YIELD: 2 servings

Ingredients

- 1 tablespoon whole-grain mustard
- 1 tablespoon lemon juice
- 1 tablespoon along with 2 tablespoon olive oil (extra virgin)
- 1/2-pound broccoli florets (torn into 2"pieces)
- 1/2-pound small red potatoes (unpeeled & halved)
- 1/2 tablespoon honey
- 2 (6oz-8oz) of center-cut without salmon fillets(1 - 1 ½"thick)
- 2 tablespoon fresh minced chives
- salt & ground black pepper for taste

Directions:

1. Set the lowest location of the toaster oven rack, pick the convection setting, and heat the oven to 500 °F.

2. Clean all over with 1 teaspoon oil and spray with 1/4 teaspoon salt and 1/4 teaspoon pepper. Dry with paper towels. Until required, refrigerate it.

3. Brush the rimmed baking sheet, with a 1 tablespoon oil toaster oven. Apply 1/2 tablespoon of

oil to the potatoes, season with salt & pepper, and place the cut side down on half of the pan.

4. Apply 1/2 tablespoon of oil to the broccoli, season with salt and pepper and place on the other half of the board. Heat until potatoes are light golden brown and broccoli on the bottom is dark brown for 22 to 24 minutes, rotating the sheet halfway while baking.

5. Meanwhile, mix the chives, mustard, honey, lemon juice, 1 tablespoon of oil left in the bowl, and make a season with the salt and pepper.

6. Keep it warm, take the sheet from the oven, and pass the bowl's broccoli. To make it browned, cover with foil. Remove any pieces of broccoli left on the sheet by using a spatula. Keep the potatoes on the pan.

7. Place the salmon skin side down on the mat and spread equally. Place the sheet in the oven and reduce the temperature of the oven to 275 °F instantly. Bake until the fillet centers reaches at 125 °F (medium-rare) for 11 to 15 minutes, turning the sheet halfway through the baking process. Move the potatoes and salmon to your broccoli platter. Serve with a dressing of chives.

5.3 Daphne Oz's Stuffed Peppers

YIELD: 3 servings

Ingredients

- 1 cup cooked wild rice, grains, quinoa & farro
- 1 tablespoon of chile powder
- 1 tablespoon of cumin
- 1/2 cup of black beans
- 1/2 cup of grated jack cheese
- 1/2-pound ground turkey
- 1-2 cups grilled veggies such as zucchini and onion (diced)
- 2 cloves minced garlic
- 3 poblano peppers (half cut & with removed seeds)
- 3 tablespoons of olive oil (divided)
- Greek yogurt (optional)

- Kosher salt and cracked black pepper, to taste
- lime wedges (optional)
- salsa (optional)
- sliced avocado (optional)

Directions:

1. First, heat the oven to 375 °F.
2. On a sheet pan lined with parchment, put the peppers and sprinkle with the olive oil and season with pepper and salt.
3. Place them in the oven and cook until tender for 15-18 minutes, but they should still retain their form. Take it out of the oven and set it aside.
4. Over a medium-high flame, heat a large skillet and add the remaining olive oil. To the pan, add the ground turkey, season with pepper and salt and all the spices. Add the garlic and cook for about five more minutes before the turkey has been browned. Remove and transfer to a wide bowl from the heat. Stir in the quinoa or the other grains, veggies, and beans on the barbecue. Taste and uniformly distribute the mixture between the peppers for seasoning.
5. Top with the cheese and put it back in the oven for another 15 minutes until the cheese melts and the entire filling is hot. On a plate, put each pepper and top with your favorite toppings.

5.4 Whole Grain Pasta & Pumpkin Bake

YIELD: 4 servings

Ingredients

- Kosher salt & cracked black pepper for taste
- 3/4-pound whole-grain penne
- 1/2 tablespoon paprika
- 1 cup toasted whole wheat bread-crumbs
- 1 clove garlic (peeled)
- 1 (15 oz)-Can of pumpkin puree (unsweetened)

- 1 (15 oz)-Can of coconut milk

Directions

1. First, heat the oven to 350°F.

2. Put a big pot to boil the water and season with salt liberally. Following the package directions, cook the pasta for 2 minutes. Reserve and set aside 2 cups of pasta water. Drain the spaghetti, put it in a mixing bowl and set it aside.

3. In a mixer, mix the coconut milk, ginger, pumpkin puree, salt and plenty of crushed black pepper. Blend until smooth, and add (if necessary) some pasta water to make it thin. The noodles drain a lot of the sauce, so it should be thin enough to easily pour from the carafe.

4. Pour over the spaghetti with the pumpkin sauce and stir to coat. Cover with bread-crumbs and put in a baking dish. Place for 15 minutes in the oven until golden brown color appears, bubbling along the edges.

5.5 Daphne Oz's Philly Cheesesteak Tacos

YIELD: 4 servings

Ingredients

- 5 button mushrooms/creminis (stemmed by caps-thinly sliced)
- 4-6 6"flour tortillas
- 2 tablespoon butter (unsalted)
- 2 tablespoon olive oil (extra virgin)
- 2 oregano sprigs/1 teaspoon dried
- 1 teaspoon of Kosher salt
- 1 thinly sliced, cored & seeded red bell pepper
- 1 lb. skirt steak
- 1 halved & thinly sliced medium onion
- 1 cup of low-moisture mozzarella/Monterey jack cheese

Directions:

1. Melt butter over medium heat in a medium skillet. Season with salt and pepper on the steak, and transfer to the pan. For medium-rare or longer, sear on both sides for 4 minutes if you want it to cook more. Take the steak out of the pan and let it sit for 10 minutes.

2. Cover the pan with 1 teaspoon of olive oil and add the oregano and onion. To caramelize the onions, simmer for 30 minutes over a low flame. Stir in the bell peppers and simmer for about 5 more minutes until they become soft.

3. Take the steak out of the pan and apply the remaining olive oil along with the mushrooms to the pan. Cook until browned and introduce salt to the seasoning.

4. Cut the steak with the mushrooms and add them to the pan. Stir in the peppers and onions. Top with the cheese and to melt, cover the plate.

5. Heat the tortillas and fill with the top. Now you can serve.

5.6 Vegetables and Turkey Stir-Fry

YIELD: 8 Servings

Ingredients

- Thin slices & minced ginger root
- 3 cups cooked brown rice
- 2 cups chopped fresh, canned or frozen vegetables such as mushrooms, bok choy, celery & water chestnuts
- 1 tablespoon oil
- 1 cup turkey (cut into ½" cubes)
- 1 peeled & minced clove garlic/1/8 tsp garlic powder
- ½ teaspoon sugar
- ½ teaspoon salt

Directions:

1. Heat the oil over medium heat in a large skillet. Add the salt, the turkey, the root of ginger, the garlic, and the vegetables. For 1 minute, please do a stir-fry. To avoid scorching, reduce the heat.

Only add sugar.

2. Remove the pan from the heat until the vegetables are tender. Add 1-2 tablespoons of water and simmer for 2 more minutes until tender or if the vegetables are still hard. Serve with rice (or noodles). Leftovers can be refrigerated within 2-3 hours.

5.7 Pantry Minestrone

YIELD: 8 servings

Ingredients

- Kosher salt & cracked black pepper for taste
- 6 cups vegetable /chicken stock (low-sodium)
- 3 tablespoons of basil pesto
- 2 tablespoons of tomato paste
- 2 tablespoons of olive oil
- 2 cups frozen (thawed) vegetable medley
- 2 cups frozen (thawed) broccoli
- 2 cloves sliced garlic
- 2 drained & rinsed-Can of white beans
- 1 sweet potato (peeled & diced)
- 1 onion (diced)
- 1 cup Spinach (frozen)
- 1 bay leaf
- 1 (28 oz) can of whole peeled tomatoes (roughly chopped)

Directions:

1. Over medium to high heat, warm up a big Dutch oven or soup pot and add olive oil. Add the onions, garlic, sweet potatoes, and season with salt and pepper when warmed.

2. Add the tomato paste and simmer for an extra 3 minutes. Add the broccoli, Spinach and veggies and cook until it gets warm. Boil and stir in the tomatoes, beans, and stock. Put the bay leaf in and

reduce the heat to a low level.

3. For 25 to 30 minutes, cook. Taste and ladle into bowls for seasoning. Using basil pesto for topping and serve with crusty bread.

5.8 Tex-Mex Loaded Baked Sweet Potatoes

YIELD: 4 Servings

Ingredients

- ¼ cup cilantro or scallions (chopped)
- ½ cup Greek yogurt / light sour cream (fat-free)
- ½ cup Mexican cheese blend (reduced fat)
- ½ cup salsa (non-compulsory)
- ½ red onion (diced about ½ cup)
- ½ teaspoon cumin
- ½ teaspoon paprika
- 1 1/3 cups of canned sodium black beans (reduced, rinsed and drained)
- 1 red pepper (diced about ½ cup)
- 1 teaspoon of chili powder
- 1 teaspoon of low sodium taco seasoning
- 1 teaspoon of olive oil
- 4 medium-sized potatoes (sweet)
- Pinch of salt

Directions:

1. Poke holes with a fork in the potato, cook on the potato setting of your microwave until the potatoes are soft and cooked through (for 4 potatoes, around 8-10 minutes on high). Cook in the oven for around 45 minutes at 400 °F, if you don't have a microwave.

2. In a shallow bowl, add the yogurt and taco seasoning and meld well.

3. Heat oil over low heat in a medium pot. Add the peppers, chili powder, onions, paprika, salt and

cumin and simmer for around 5 minutes until the onions are gently caramelized.

4. Now include black beans and mix to blend and heat (approximately for 5 more minutes).

5. Cut down the potato lengthwise or use a fork to pierce the surface.

6. Cover with 1/3 cup of black bean blend, 2 tablespoons of shredded cheese, 2 tablespoons of Greek yogurt blend and 2 tablespoons of salsa.

5.9 Tandoori Chicken

YIELD: 6 Servings

Ingredients

- 6 boneless, skinless chicken breasts (cut into 1-2" pieces)
- 6 skewers (soaked in water, at least for 15 minutes)
- 5 crushed garlic cloves
- 2 tablespoon paprika
- 1 teaspoon yellow curry powder
- 1 teaspoon ground ginger
- 1 teaspoon red pepper flakes - crushed (use ½ teaspoon for a milder flavor)
- 1 cup plain yogurt (nonfat)
- ½ cup lemonade

Directions:

1. 1st heat the oven to 400 °F. In a blender, combine the milk, garlic, lemon juice, ginger, yellow curry powder, red pepper flakes and paprika and mix smoothly.
2. Onto each of the soaked skewers, skewer the equivalent number of chicken bits. Place the chicken skewers in a shallow casserole dish. Add half of a mixture of yogurt, and reserved the rest. Cover for about 15 minutes and cool.
3. With cooking sauce, spray another small baking dish. Remove the chicken skewers, dispose of the marinade with the yogurt, and put the chicken skewers in the bowl. Brush the chicken with a blend of reserved yogurt.
4. Bake for 15-20 minutes or until juices run clear when meat is pierced. Instantly serve. Grill the

chicken, skewers over medium-high heat for 3-5 minutes on either hand for much more authentic preparation.

5.10 Turkey Fajitas Bowls

YIELD: 4 Servings

Ingredients

- 4 tablespoons salsa (for topping)
- 4- 8 inches corn tortillas (or you can make your particular tostada bowls)
- 3/4 tsp fresh chile pepper or dried for taste
- 2 tsp olive oil
- 1/2 tsp dried oregano leaves
- 1/2 lb. turkey breast
- 1/2 large piece yellow bell pepper (cut into 1"piece)
- 1/2 big green pepper (cut into 1"piece)
- 1/2 cup cheddar cheese (shredded) for topping
- 1 tbsp lemon juice
- 1 medium tomato (pierce into 12 wedges)
- 1 crushed clove Garlic

Directions:

1. Tear the turkey into thin slices and then into 3/4-inch short strips. Add 1 tablespoon of oil with garlic, lemon juice, oregano and chili pepper in a medium dish. Add the turkey and stir for coating. Let it marinate for half an hour.

2. Heat the remaining 1 tbsp oil in a nonstick skillet at medium-high heat. Stir in the yellow and green peppers and fry for 2 minutes. Add the turkey strips and fry for an extra 3 minutes. Heat the tomatoes and stir.

3. In a pan, hot tortillas are used as a basis. Pour in the bowl of tortilla or tostada and top with salsa and cheese.

5.11 Sesame-Honey Chicken & Quinoa Bowl

YIELD: 4 Servings

Ingredients

Quinoa and carrot slaw:

- 3/4 cup quinoa, rinsed
- 1 & 1/2 cup water
- 2 cups of grated carrots (approximately 3 large)
- 2 tbsp rice vinegar
- 2 tbsp toasted sesame seeds
- 1 tbsp sesame oil

Sesame-Honey Chicken:

- 3 tablespoons reduced-sodium soy sauce
- 3 tablespoons honey
- 2 tablespoons water
- 2 tbsp sesame oil
- 2 scallions (sliced)
- 2 cups prepared chicken breast (pierce into the bite-sized pieces)
- 1 teaspoon cornstarch

Directions:

1. To make the quinoa: Boil 1½ cups of water in a shallow saucepan. Add the quinoa and put it to a boil again. Reduce to a medium boil, cover and cook for 10 to 14 minutes before the water is absorbed. Uncover them and wait.

2. Meanwhile, in a medium dish, mix the rice vinegar, carrots, rice vinegar, seeds, sesame and 1 tablespoon of the oil. Put it aside.

3. Combine the soy sauce, sesame oil, sugar, and cornstarch 2 teaspoons of water in a shallow cup. Pour it into a medium skillet. Cook and stir over medium heat until the sauce becomes thickened. Add the chicken and stir for about 1 minute before it is coated with the sauce.

4. Divide the quinoa and top each with 1/2 cup of carrot slaw and 3/4 cup of chicken mixture in 4 cups. Sprinkle with green onion.

5.12 Southwest Tortilla Bake

YIELD: 4 Servings

Ingredients

- Salsa
- Eight corn tortillas (cut in half)
- 3 eggs
- 2 green onions (sliced)
- 1/2 tsp chili powder
- 1 tomato (sliced)
- 1 cup Monterey Jack cheese (shredded)
- 1 cup fresh / frozen corn
- 1 cup milk (fat-free)
- 1 cup of cooked black / pinto beans
- 1 4-ounce can green chilies (diced)

Directions:

1. 1st heat the oven up to 350 °F.

2. Using nonstick spray or oil to coat an 8-inch square baking dish. Arrange 5 tortilla halves to line the bottom of the plate. Top each of cheese, corn and beans with 1/3 of a cup. Utilize 1/2 of the green onions to sprinkle. To layer and top with beans, 1/3 cup cheese, the leftover corn, and green onions, place a further 5 tortilla halves on top. To shield, place the last 5 tortilla pieces over the corner.

3. Add the eggs, chili powder and milk to a medium bowl and whisk to mix. Stir in the chilies. Pour the egg and milk mixture equally over the tortillas. Top with both the 1/3 cup of left cheese and tomato slices.

4. Uncovered and bake for about 50 minutes until a knife inserted in the middle. Let it stand at

room temperature for 10 minutes before serving. Serve hot with salsa.

5.13 Quick Chili

YIELD: 7 Servings

Ingredients

- 1 15.5-ounces-Can of kidney beans (drained)
- 1 14.5 ounces-Can of tomatoes with liquid (diced)
- 1/2-pound lean ground meat
- 1/2 medium onion (chopped)
- 1 1/2 tbsp chili powder

Directions:

1. Over medium-high heat, onions and brown meat in a large skillet (350 degrees Fahrenheit in an electric skillet). Drain the fat.

2. Add beans, chili powder and tomatoes.

3. Reduce the heat to low (in an electric skillet at 250 degrees Fahrenheit), cover and simmer for 10 minutes.

4. Serve it hot.

5. Leftovers can be refrigerated within 2-3 hours.

5.14 Sesame Encrusted Baked Chicken Tenders

YIELD: 4 Servings

Ingredients

- olive oil spray
- 6 tablespoons sesame seeds (toasted)
- 4 tbsp panko bread-crumbs (without adding the salt)
- 2 tsp sesame oil
- 2 teaspoons soy sauce (low sodium)

- 16-ounces chicken tenderloins
- ½ tsp coarse salt

Directions:

1. Preheat to above 425 degrees Fahrenheit and spray with parchment paper or nonstick oil spray on a baking sheet.

2. In a dish, mix the soy sauce and sesame oil. In another dish, combine the panko, sesame seeds and salt.

3. Put the chicken with the soy sauce and oil in the dish, then in the mixture with sesame seeds to coat properly.

4. Place this on the baking sheet and gently spray with oil spray on the top of the chicken and bake for 8-10 minutes. Switch over and simmer for 4-5 more minutes or until it is cooked through.

5.15 Shepherd's Pie

YIELD: 6 Servings

Ingredients

- 2 bulky baking potatoes (peeled & diced)
- 1 lb. lean ground beef
- 1 medium onion (chopped)
- 1 clove garlic (minced)
- ½ cup & 2 tablespoons flour
- 4 cups of frozen vegetables (mixed)
- ground pepper for taste
- 1/2 cup milk (low-fat)
- 1/2 cup cheddar cheese (shredded)
- 3/4 cup beef broth (reduced sodium)

Directions:

1. In a saucepan, put the diced potatoes and add enough water to barely cover. Just bring it to a

boil. Diminish the heat and simmer, and covered it until soft (around 15 minutes).

2. Drain and mash the potatoes. Add milk and set aside the mixture.

3. Preheat the oven to 375 °C.

4. Put brown meat, garlic and onion in a large skillet. Stir in the flour. Cook and constantly stir for 1 minute.

5. Add the broth and vegetables. Cook for five minutes until it's bubbly. Just stir well.

6. Spoon the mixture of vegetables into an 8-inch square baking dish. Spread the mixture of potatoes over the vegetable/meat mixture. Sprinkle the cheese.

7. Bake for 25 minutes, until bubbly and hot.

8. Within 2-3 hours, refrigerate the leftovers.

Chapter 6 – Dessert

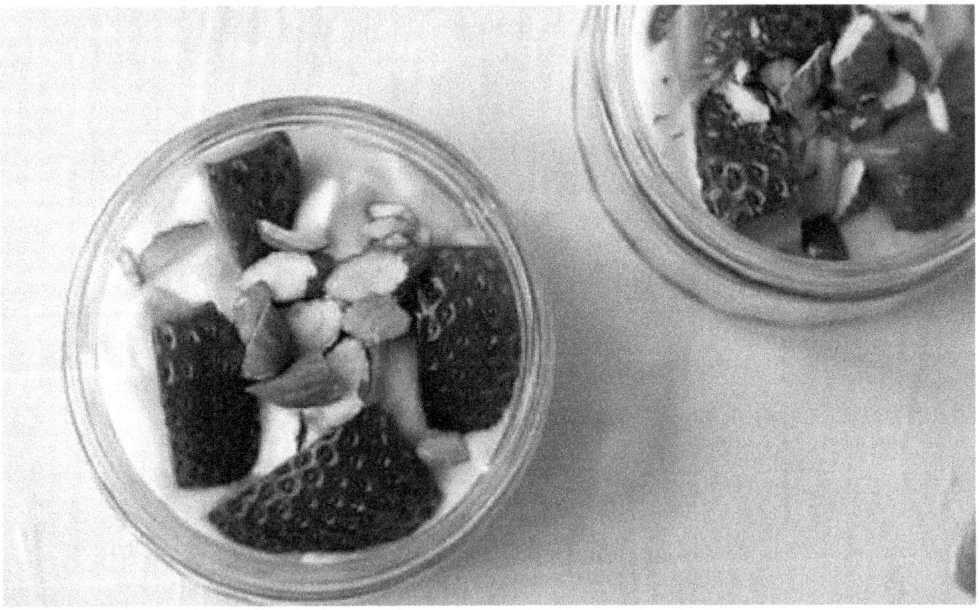

6.1 Gail Simmons' Cherry Vanilla Float

YIELD: 2 servings

Ingredients

- club soda/seltzer (chilled)
- vanilla ice cream
- whole frozen (thawed) pitted cherries for serving
- 2-1/2 cups of frozen dark cherries (pitted & finely chopped)
- 1/2 teaspoon crudely ground black pepper
- 2 tablespoon sugar
- 1/8 teaspoon pure vanilla extract

Directions

For the syrup:

1. In a shallow saucepan, combine the sliced cherries, cinnamon, pepper, salt and 3/4 of a water cup.
2. Bring over medium heat to an active boil and cook until it has a dense syrup consistency (around 15 minutes).

3. Strain the syrup into a bowl using a fine-mesh strainer, softly but tightly pressing on the solids and scraping the strainer's bottom to remove much syrup as feasible and discard the solids.
4. Stir in vanilla and cool thoroughly for 15 to 20 minutes. Makes 2/3 of a cup.

To make the float:

In an 8-ounce bottle, apply 2 teaspoons syrup and finish with 1/2 cup cold club soda. Attach an ice cream scoop and decorate with a few entire cherries.

6.2 Gail Simmons' Roasted Banana, Chocolate, Whole Wheat-Quinoa Bread

YIELD: 10 servings

Ingredients

- 1 teaspoon baking soda
- 2 tablespoon sugar
- 2 large eggs
- 4 bananas (3 coarsely mashed & 1 thin sliced lengthwise)
- 2 tablespoon yogurt
- 1 teaspoon pure vanilla extract
- 1/2 teaspoon cinnamon
- 1/2 cup of vegetable oil (for greasing pan)
- 1/2 cup of dark chocolate chips
- 1/4 teaspoon Kosher salt
- 3/4 cup and tablespoon whole wheat flour
- 3/4 cup of quinoa flour

Directions:

1. Preheat the oven to 350 degrees Fahrenheit. Oil a loaf pan generously, then sprinkle with 2 teaspoons of whole wheat flour and remove the extra flour.

2. Whisk together the whole wheat, baking soda, quinoa flour, cinnamon and salt in a bowl.

3. Whisk the sugar and eggs together in a separate bowl until smooth. In a slow stream, add milk, whisk until combined, then mix in the mashed bananas, vanilla and yogurt. Fold gently in the combination of flour and chocolate to mix.

4. In the prepared loaf pan, add the batter and finish with the remaining banana slices.

5. Bake for about 45 minutes until the bread becomes golden and then inject the wooden skewer in the middle to clean.

6. Cool the loaf for about 10 minutes in a pan on a wire rack, then switch on the rack. Turn the right side of the loaf up to allow slightly more cooling before slicing. Serve at room temperature or warm.

6.3 Heart Healthy Chocolate Chip Cookies

YIELD: 24 SERVINGS

Ingredients

- 4 tablespoon butter substitute
- 2 cups of rolled oats
- 1/4 teaspoon baking soda
- 1/3 cup dried cranberries
- 1/2 teaspoon salt
- 1/2 cup tahini
- 1/2 cup walnuts (chopped)
- 1 large egg
- 1 cup cacao chocolate chips (60%)
- 1-1/4 cups of whole wheat flour
- 1-1/4 cups of brown rice syrup
- 1-1/2 teaspoon vanilla extract
- 1-1/2 teaspoon cinnamon

Directions:

1. Preheat the oven to 375 °F. Cover a sheet of parchment paper for baking.
2. In a cup, whisk in the flour, oats, cinnamon, salt and baking soda. Beat the tahini and butter substitute in a mixer bowl until it is smooth. Mix in the brown rice syrup and beat until well mixed, at low speed. Beat the egg and vanilla at low speed until blended. Fold in the chocolate chips, walnuts and cranberries with a spatula when mixed.
3. On a baking sheet, drop a tablespoon of dough. Slightly flatten the dough with a fingertip. Place the dough on a cookie sheet approximately 2 inches apart. Bake for about 10-11 minutes, until it is light brown.
4. Enable to cool for 5 minutes on the baking sheet before removing.

6.4 Blueberry Bling

YIELD: 4 Servings

Ingredients

- 3 cups fresh/frozen blueberries
- 2 teaspoons butter or margarine (soft salted)
- 1 tablespoon of brown sugar
- 1 tablespoon of all-purpose flour
- ½ teaspoon cinnamon
- ½ cup oats (rolled)

Direction:

1. Preheat the oven to 375 °C.
2. Clean the blueberries, rinse them, and put them on a 9-inch pie plate.
3. Mix the butter, sugar, oatmeal, flour and cinnamon in a small bowl with a fork. Sprinkle over the blueberries with the oat mixture.
4. Bake for roughly 25 minutes. Enjoy while it is hot.

6.5 Fabulous Fig Bars

YIELD: **24** Servings

Ingredients

- 1-1/4 cups oats (old fashioned rolled)
- 1/3 cup sugar
- 1/2 cup walnuts (chopped)
- 1/4 cup of orange juice (juice from 1/2 orange)
- 1/2 cup margarine/butter (softened)
- 1-1/2 cups of all-purpose flour
- 1/2 teaspoon of baking soda
- 16-ounces dried figs (stemmed chopped)
- 2 Tablespoons of hot water
- 1 cup of packed brown sugar
- 1 large egg

Directions:

1. Preheat oven to 350 degrees. Lightly spray or oil a 9x13-inch baking pan.
2. Combine the figs, walnuts, sugar, orange juice and hot water in a mixing bowl and set aside.
3. Mix margarine and brown sugar until creamy. Add egg and mix until smooth.
4. Mix flour and baking soda. Stir into the egg mixture. Blend in oats to make a soft dough.
5. Reserve 1 cup of dough for topping. With floured fingertips, press the remaining dough into a thin layer on the bottom of the baking pan.
6. Spread fig mixture evenly over the dough. Crumble reserved dough over the top, allowing fig mixture to show.
7. Bake 30 minutes or until golden brown. Cool completely in baking pan. Cut into 24 bars (about 2.5 x 2 inches).

6.6 Whoopie Pies

YIELD: 5 serving

Ingredients

For the cake:

- ¼ cup vegetable shortening
- ½ teaspoon of pure vanilla extract
- 1 large egg
- 1 large egg white (pasteurized)
- 1 package 18.25-ounces mixed plain chocolate cake
- 2 cups sifted confectioners' sugar
- 8 tablespoons butter (melted)

Directions:

1. Making of cakes: In the center of the oven, put a rack and preheat the oven to 350 °F. Place 2 unoiled baking sheets aside.

2. In a large mixing bowl, put the cake mix, egg and butter and beat with an electric mixer at low speed for 1 to 2 minutes until the ingredients come together in a stiff mass. Using your hands, form the dough into 1-inch balls or scoop the dough into balls. Place the dough balls on baking sheets that are 2 inches away.

3. keep baking sheets in an oven and bake up cakes for 10 to 12 minutes until they are still slightly soft. If your oven can not accommodate both baking sheets on the center rack, put one on the top rack and one on the center rack and rotate them halfway through the baking time. Take the baking sheets from the oven and cool for 5 minutes with the cakes on them. Then move the cakes to wire racks using a metal spatula to cool fully, for 30 minutes longer.

5. Make the filling: Put the sugar, egg white, shortening, and vanilla of the confectioners in a medium-sized mixing bowl and beat at low speed with an electric mixer until it is mixed in 1 minute. Spoon about 1 teaspoon onto one cake's flat foot. To make a sandwich, cover the filling with a second cake. Repeat and serve with the remaining cakes.

6.7 Spaghetti Pie

YIELD: 3 servings

Ingredients:

- 3 large eggs
- 2 tablespoon of olive oil
- 12 oz. spaghetti (Reserve half cup of water for later)
- 1 yellow onion (chopped)
- 1 teaspoon of Chia Seeds
- 1 tablespoon dry mixed herbs (3 tbsp of fresh)
- 1 pound of ground turkey/chicken or beef)
- 1 cup of tomato paste
- 1 cup - 2% of shredded mozzarella
- 1 cup - 2% of grated Parmesan cheese
- ½ red capsicums
- ½ green capsicums

Directions:

1. Preheat the oven to 350 °F.
2. Sauté the onions in a large skillet until tender. Add beef or ground turkey and 3⁄4 cup of tomato paste. Apply half of the pasta water and stir well with the capsicums and chia seeds.
3. Add more boiling water if needed, but consistency should be like a thick Bolognese sauce.
4. Mix the cooked pasta, parmesan cheese, eggs, 1⁄4 cup of the tomato paste and 1 cup of mozzarella in a wide dish.
5. Use the olive oil on a 9 or 10-inch pie pan.
6. Spread over the bottom of the cooking pan with the half beef mixture. To level it, apply the spaghetti mixture and press to make it flat.
7. Spread the leftover mozzarella on top, along with the remaining meat mixture.

8. Bake the pastry for 30 to 35 minutes in the oven. Please pick from the oven and leave it for about 10 minutes. Make slices with a sharp knife or pizza slicer, similar to a pie. Use a green salad while serving.

6.8 Amazing Ate-Layer Dip

YIELD: 8 servings

Ingredients

- 1 cup heated canned black beans
- 1 cup onion (diced)
- 1 ounce of Galaxy Veggie Shreds (Cheddar/another low-calorie cheese)
- 1 pouch - 4 ounces BOCA Ground Burger/another ground meat's substitute, such as Morningstar Farms version
- 10 ounces butternut squash cubes (around 2 and 1/2 cups)
- 2 cups of chopped cherry tomatoes
- 3-1/2 teaspoon of taco seasoning
- 4 cups of shredded lettuce
- 4 ounces of fat-free sour cream
- 4 ounces chopped roasted red peppers (shouldn't be packed in oil)
- lime juice, pepper & salt (Optional)

Directions:

1. Start by mixing half of the tomatoes and all the onions. Season with lime juice, salt and pepper to taste, if necessary and keep aside.
2. Then, nuke the squash with 2 tablespoons of water for 6 to 7 minutes in a sealed microwave-safe dish (until squash is soft enough to mash). Mash the squash to a pulp using a fork or a potato masher. Combine the 1-1/2 teaspoons. Season with the taco and put aside.
3. Combine the tomatoes and Boca Ground Burger and the leftover 2 tsp of taco seasoning in a skillet sprayed with nonstick spray and cook until the crumbles are defrosted, and the mixture is fully heated.

4. Place items in the following order in a broad dish: lettuce, blended tomato and onion, butternut squash, sour cream, beef blend, black beans, cheese shreds and red peppers. Serve the delicious (hot or cold).

6.9 Tomato Spinach Chicken Spaghetti

Servings: 4 servings

Ingredients

- 8-oz. fresh spinach
- 8-oz. spaghetti pasta
- 4 chopped Roma tomatoes
- 3 tablespoons of olive oil (use the high quality/oil extracted from the sun-dried tomatoes)
- 3 chopped garlic cloves
- 2 tablespoons of olive oil (drained from sun-dried tomatoes)
- 1/4 teaspoon salt
- 1/4 teaspoon salt
- 1/4 teaspoon of red pepper flakes
- 1/4 cup of sun-dried tomatoes (drained of oil)
- 1/4 cup of chopped fresh basil leaves
- 1/2 pound chopped boneless and skinless chicken (if possible, boneless and skinless thighs)

Directions:

1. On medium-low heat, add the sliced sun-dried tomatoes and 2 tablespoons of the olive oil drained from the sun-dried tomatoes to a large skillet.
2. Add a chicken (chopped) if possible; use the boneless and skinless chicken thighs, but you may also use minced chicken breast.
3. In the skillet, sprinkle red pepper flakes and salt to all the ingredients.
4. Cook for about 5 minutes on medium heat until the chicken is fully cooked and no longer pink.
5. Cover the chicken skillet with chopped fresh basil leaves, chopped tomatoes, chopped garlic

and fresh spinach. Cook for around 3-5 minutes on medium heat until the spinach wilts and tomatoes secrete some of their juices. Retract from the heat.

6. Taste it, and if necessary, add more salt for taste. Close the lid to hold the heat off.
7. Following the packet instructions, cook the pasta and drain it.
8. With the vegetable and chicken, add the fried and drained pasta to the skillet.
9. Reheat at low temperature, blend properly and add more seasonings, if desired (salt and pepper). Withdraw from the sun.

You may add more high-quality olive oil at this stage while the pasta and vegetables are off-heat. It's not mandatory but is delicious indeed. Alternatively, you can apply more olive oil from the sun-dried tomato container.

6.10 Yogurt with Fresh Strawberries and Honey

YIELD: 1 serving

Ingredients:

- 4 teaspoons of honey
- 4 Tablespoons of toasted sliced almonds
- 3 cups of plain low-fat yogurt
- 1-pint strawberries (fresh)

Directions:

1. Clean and carve the strawberries into pieces and keep on side.
2. Put 3/4 cups of yogurt in each of the 4 serving plates. Divide the strawberries equally between the plates. Top each with 1 teaspoon of honey along with the topping of 1 tablespoon of toasted sliced almonds. Instantly serve now.

6.11 Pear-Cranberry Pie with Oatmeal Streusel

YIELD: 2 servings

Ingredients:

Streusel:

- 1/3 light brown sugar (packed)
- 1 tbsp unsalted butter (Chilled and small pieces)
- ¾ cup of regular oats
- ½ teaspoon of ground cinnamon
- ¼ teaspoon of ground nutmeg

Filling:

- ½ cup light brown sugar (packed)
- 2 ½ tablespoons of cornstarch
- 2 cups of fresh cranberries
- 3 cups (a half-inch) cubed (peeled /unpeeled) and 2 large pears

Remaining ingredient:

- 1 9"deep-dish pie crust (unbaked)

Directions:

1. Preheat the oven to 350 °F.
2. Combine the first 4 ingredients in a medium bowl to cook streusel; cut into butter with a pastry cutter or 2 knives till the mixture is comparable to a coarse meal.
3. Combine cranberries, 2/3 cup of brown sugar, corn starch and pear in a wide bowl to prepare the filling. So mix well to combine. Sprinkle streusel over pear mixture and spoon the pear mixture into pastry shell.
4. Cook for 1 hour at 350 degrees or it is creamy, and streusel is browned. Cool it on a wire rack for at least 1 hour.

Chapter 7 – Appetizer

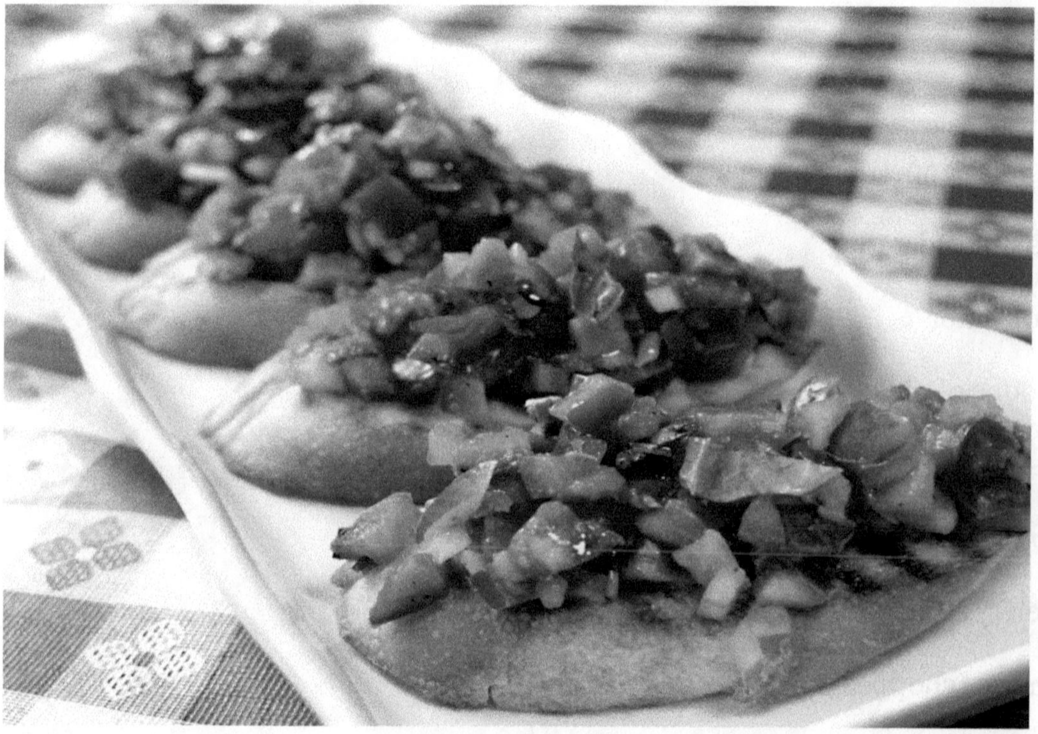

7.1 Chef Roblé Ali's Homemade Guacamole

YIELD: 4 servings

Ingredients

- pinch of cumin
- pinch of coriander
- pinch of chili powder
- 2 avocados
- 1/4 cup scallions (chopped)
- 1/2 cup tomatoes (diced)
- 1 caustic lime (cut in half)
- 1 clove garlic (chopped)

Directions:

1. Scoop and mash the avocado into a bowl.
2. Add other ingredients and mix well and serve.

7.2 Vegetable Pasta Soup

YIELD: 3 servings

Ingredients

- 12 (3/4-cup) appetizer servings
- 6 cloves minced garlic
- 4 cups of water
- 2 teaspoons of olive oil
- 2 tablespoons fresh parsley (snipped)
- 1/4 cup Parmesan cheese (shaved)
- 1 cup celery (thinly sliced)
- 1 cup onion (chopped)
- 1 32-ounce box chicken broth (reduced-sodium)
- 1 1/2 cups ditalini pasta (dried)
- 1 1/2 cups coarsen carrot (shredded)

Directions:

1. Heat the oil over medium heat in a 5 to 6 quart Dutch oven. Combine with garlic; simmer for 15 seconds. Add the onion, carrot, and celery and then roast and stir regularly for 5 -7 min until it is tender. Add the water and chicken broth and allow it to boil. Stir in uncooked pasta and boil for 7 - 8 mins or until it is tender.
2. Cover individual pieces of parsley and Parmesan cheese to eat. Allows 12 servings of (3/4-cup) appetizer.

7.3 Jamika Pessoa's Thai Peanut Salad

YIELD: 4 SERVINGS

Ingredients

- Kosher salt & black pepper (cracked)
- juice & zest (half a lime)

- 3 tablespoons of soy sauce
- 3 scallions (sliced)
- 2 tablespoon water (if needed to thin)
- 2 tablespoon rice or apple cider vinegar
- 1/4 cup lumpy peanut butter
- 1/2 teaspoon fresh/ground ginger
- 1/2 cup of cilantro leaves
- 1 tablespoon honey
- 1 cup chicken (shredded)
- 1 bag cabbage and carrot mix (shredded)

Directions

1. Put the cabbage in a serving bowl with the scallions, carrots, cilantro and chicken.
2. In a small cup, combine the remaining ingredients and whisk until combined.
3. Over the salad, pour the dressing and serve.

7.4 Bruschetta

YIELD: 2 servings

Ingredients:

- Parmesan Cheese (low fat)
- 3 tomatoes (diced)
- 2 tsp balsamic vinegar
- 2 tbsp basil (chopped)
- 2 cloves garlic (minced)
- 1/2 whole-grain bread (cut into six ½" thick diagonal pieces)
- 1 tsp olive oil
- 1 tsp black pepper

- 1 tbsp chopped parsley

Directions:

1. Toast flatbread slices until finely browned in an oven at 400 °F.
2. Mix it with all of the rest of the ingredients.
3. Blend the spoon equally over the toasted bread.
4. Topping with a little Parmesan egg.
5. Serve it while it is warm.

Conclusion

The risks of having high blood pressure or hypertension are determined by what you choose to eat.

Along with therapeutic intervention and behavioral improvements, the DASH diet seemed to be successful. In several clinical trials, the DASH diet has been well studied and found in lowering the blood pressure. DASH diet has been prescribed as the safest diet for those who wish to lose weight and reduce blood pressure. For optimal management of elevated BP, the DASH eating pattern (like other lifestyle interventions) is significant. Behavioral modifications are most commonly prescribed along with anti-hypertensive drugs, although they are regarded as a pillar of treatment.

So along with the use of the DASH diet, life changes should be in consideration. The DASH diet contains fruits, whole grains, vegetables, low-fat dairy products, fish, lean meats, and lessened sugar-sweetened desserts and some drinks that successfully decrease BP alone and in tandem with other medications. The rise in fruits and vegetables improves the diet's potassium and calcium content. DASH diet focus on lowering dietary sodium and promoting the consumption of calcium, potassium, and magnesium.

There is also evidence that the DASH diet has minimized the risk of cardiovascular heart disease, stroke, type 2 diabetes, and obesity. While vigilance should be exercised in patients with Chronic Kidney Disease (CKD), Diabetes mellitus (DM), Cardiovascular Disease (CVD), or recommended RAAS (Renin-Angiotensin-Aldosterone System) inhibitors, patient.

Therefore, for particular nutrients such as sodium, potassium, calcium, and food eaten by the population, country-specific dietary guidelines are required. In addition, for public health and clinical research, empirical studies to define the temporal correlations between the use of DASH diets and its impact on blood pressure are too essential.

Unfortunately, the diet's conformity remains poor. Studies on the long-term effectiveness of the DASH diet remain outside of clinical trials. Further research should be put on exploring the benefits of the DASH diet. Health care teams should be aware of playing their role in educating the patients about this diet's effects.

CPSIA information can be obtained
at www.ICGtesting.com
Printed in the USA
LVHW100953180121
676360LV00039B/930